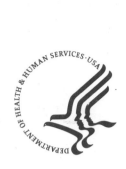

ORI

Introduction to the Responsible Conduct of Research

Nicholas H. Steneck
illustrations by David Zinn

Updated Edition
August 2007

US GOVERNMENT OFFICIAL EDITION NOTICE

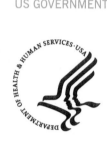

Legal Status and Use of Seals and Logos

The seal of the U.S. Department of Health and Human Services (HHS) authenticates this publication as the Official U.S. Government edition of the *ORI Introduction to the Responsible Conduct of Research*.

Under the provisions of 42 U.S.C. 132b-10, the unauthorized use of this seal in a publication is prohibited and subject to a civil penalty of up to $5,000 for each unauthorized copy of it that is reprinted or distributed.

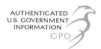

USE of ISBN Prefix

This is the Official U.S. Government edition of this publication and is herein identified to certify its authenticity. Use of the 978-0-16-072285-1 ISBN is for this U.S. Government Printing Office Official Edition only. The Superintendent of Documents of the U.S. Government Printing Office requests that any reprinted edition be labeled clearly as a copy of the authentic work with a new ISBN.

Disclaimer

The *ORI Introduction to the Responsible Conduct of Research* is not an official policy statement or guideline and should not be viewed as such. While every effort has been made to present an accurate description of Federal rules and the practices accepted by the research community for the responsible conduct of research, any statement in this *ORI Introduction to RCR* that is inconsistent with Federal law or regulation or official policy or guidance is superseded thereby. This document is also not intended to create any right or benefit, substantive or procedural, enforceable at law by a party against the United States, its agencies, officers, or employees or any PHS-funded research institution or its officers, employees, or research staff.

Copyright and Acknowledgment Notice

ORI requests that any re-use or re-publication of any of the materials contained within the *ORI Introduction to the Responsible Conduct of Research* acknowledge the source. Copyright for the illustrations appearing herein is held by the artist, David Zinn. Limited personal and educational use of these illustrations is permitted with appropriate attribution to the artist. Inquiries regarding other uses of the illustrations should be addressed to the artist at dszinn@umich.edu. Other questions about re-use and re-publication should be addressed to askori@hhs.gov.

Message from the Secretary of Health and Human Services

Advances in scientific knowledge have provided the foundation for improvements in public health and have led to enhanced health and quality of life for all Americans. Many of these advances can be traced to the work of the U.S. Department of Health and Human Services (HHS), which supports the world's largest medical research effort.

Research conducted with support from HHS also helps to assure the safety of foods and health care products, is vital in the fight against drug and alcohol abuse, and in many other ways fosters the Department's mission to improve health and to help those in need of assistance.

As the custodian of the largest share of our Nation's resources devoted to biomedical and behavioral research, HHS takes seriously the challenge of ensuring these resources are used responsibly. Special programs already exist to oversee the protection of human and animal subjects in research, to review conflicts of interest, and to assure laboratory safety and responsible grants management.

With this publication, we hope to encourage researchers and research institutions to make a special effort to understand, discuss, and teach others about the responsible conduct of research.

Tommy S. Thompson

Tommy G. Thompson
Secretary
U.S. Department of Health and Human Services
2001-2005

Foreword

The Office of Research Integrity (ORI) oversees and directs Public Health Service (PHS) research integrity activities on behalf of the Secretary of Health and Human Services and the American public. This responsibility extends to around $30 billion in Federal research support, devoted primarily to the biomedical and behavioral sciences through intramural and extramural programs, and to the thousands of researchers, research staff, and research administrators who work on PHS-funded research.

As part of its efforts to promote integrity in PHS-funded research, ORI is authorized to undertake activities and to support programs that enhance education in the responsible conduct of research (RCR). The *ORI Introduction to the Responsible Conduct of Research* is being issued to further this important mission.

The importance of formal RCR education was first explicitly recognized in the 1989 Institute of Medicine Report, *The Responsible Conduct of Research in the Health Sciences*, and has since been endorsed by other groups and members of the research community. Thanks to this support, researchers who want to learn about or help others understand responsible conduct in research have many resources available, from formal courses to web-based instruction programs, a growing array of challenging books, and the experience of established researchers conveyed through mentoring.

The *ORI Introduction to RCR* seeks to supplement existing resources by making a comprehensive overview of basic rules of the road for responsible research available to all PHS-funded researchers. It has been prepared with the needs of small and mid-size research institutions and beginning researchers in mind, since we have often been asked to provide resources for this community, but it may find use in other settings.

In issuing this publication, it needs to be stressed that ORI is not establishing or even recommending how RCR ought to be taught. We understand that responsible conduct in research can be and is learned in different ways, that the standards for responsible conduct can vary from field to field, and that in many situations two or more responses to a question about responsible research may be considered acceptable research practice. We hope the *ORI Introduction to RCR* will therefore be seen as the beginning and not the end of learning about this important aspect of professional life.

Chris B. Pascal, J.D.
Director
Office of Research Integrity

Contents

Preface

Spurred by a growing belief in the importance of science and technology, public support for research increased dramatically over the course of the 20th century. A century ago, research did not play a major role in the average person's life. Today, few aspects of life are not touched in one way or another by the information and technologies generated through research.

With growing public support for research has come an understandable concern about the way it is conducted. Public funds support roughly one-third of all research and development (R&D) in the U.S. and half of all basic research. Many researchers, therefore, spend a significant portion of their time working for the public. As public servants and also professionals, researchers have clear obligations to conduct their research in a responsible manner.

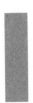

> **In general terms, responsible conduct in research is simply good citizenship applied to professional life.**

In general terms, responsible conduct in research is simply good citizenship applied to professional life. Researchers who report their work honestly, accurately, efficiently, and objectively are on the right road when it comes to responsible conduct. Anyone who is dishonest, knowingly reports inaccurate results, wastes funds, or allows personal bias to influence scientific findings is not.

However, the specifics of good citizenship in research can be a challenge to understand and put into practice. Research is not an organized profession in the same way as law or medicine. Researchers learn best practices in a number of ways and in different settings. The norms for responsible conduct can vary from field to field. Add to this the growing body of local, state, and Federal regulations and you have a situation that can test the professional savvy of any researcher.

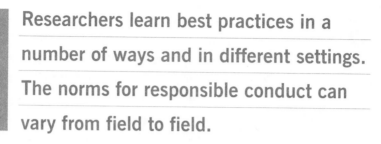

Researchers learn best practices in a number of ways and in different settings. The norms for responsible conduct can vary from field to field.

The *ORI Introduction to the Responsible Conduct of Research* has been written primarily for researchers and research staff engaged in research supported by the Public Health Service but is applicable to scholarly research in general. As an "introduction," it seeks to provide a practical overview of the rules, regulations, and professional practices that define the responsible conduct of research. The coverage is not exhaustive and leaves room for continued reading and discussion in the laboratory and classroom, at professional meetings, and in any other setting where researchers gather to discuss their work.

The content is organized around two ways of thinking about research. The main sections follow the normal flow of research, from a consideration of shared values to planning, conducting, reporting, and reviewing. The chapters within the main sections cover nine core instructional areas that have been widely recognized as central to the responsible conduct of research. An opening chapter on rules of the road and a brief epilogue on responsible research round out the coverage.

Although designed to follow the normal flow of research, the chapters in this volume are all more-or-less self-contained and can be read in any order. Each opens with a short case in which students and researchers are faced with making decisions about the responsible conduct of research. Throughout

(i) the chapters, important points are summarized in bulleted lists (✓) or noted in the margins (see left). Each chapter ends with a set of closing questions for further discussion (**1** , **2** ...) and resources for reference and additional reading. The Web addresses given for the resources and elsewhere in this work were current at the time of printing.

While written with all researchers in mind, special consideration has been given to the needs of students, postdocs, and researchers who do not have easy access to responsible conduct of research materials or to colleagues who can explain the intricacies of responsible conduct in research to them. Two or three hours with this book should provide anyone in this position with a better understanding of the reasons for and the scope of the most important responsibilities researchers have.

Many colleagues have generously provided comments on parts or all of this work as it took shape over several drafts, including Ruth Bulger, Tony Demsey, Peggy Fischer, Carolyn Fassi, Nelson Garnett, Shirley Hicks, Erich Jensen, Mike Kalichman and his students, Nell Kriesberg, John Krueger, Tony Mazzaschi, Judy Nowack, Chris Pascal, Ken Pimple, Larry Rhoades, Fran Sanden, Mary Scheetz, Joan Schwartz, David Shore, Peggy Sundermeyer, and Carol Wigglesworth. Co-creator, artist David Zinn, patiently produced multiple versions of his drawings as we worked together to turn serious dilemmas into lighter but thought-provoking illustrations. ORI Director, Chris Pascal, and Associate Director, Larry Rhoades, deserve credit for initiating and carrying through on this project. If through promoting integrity and responsible conduct in research this work helps preserve the place of research in society today, it will have been a project well worth undertaking.

Nicholas H. Steneck
Ann Arbor, MI

Part I.

Shared Values

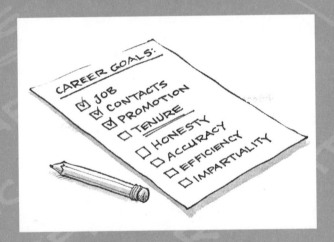

Part I: Shared Values

THERE IS NO ONE BEST WAY TO UNDERTAKE

research, no universal method that applies

to all scientific investigations. Accepted

practices for the responsible conduct of

research can and do vary from

discipline to discipline and even

from laboratory to laboratory. There

are, however, some important shared values

for the responsible conduct of research that

bind all researchers together, such as:

✓ **HONESTY** —— conveying information truthfully and honoring commitments,

✓ **ACCURACY** —— reporting findings precisely and taking care to avoid errors,

✓ **EFFICIENCY** —— using resources wisely and avoiding waste, and

✓ **OBJECTIVITY** —— letting the facts speak for themselves and avoiding improper bias.

At the very least, responsible research is research that is built on a commitment to these and other important values that define what is meant by integrity in research.

The opening chapters of the *ORI Introduction to RCR* provide a framework for thinking about basic values in the context of the day-to-day practice of research.

Chapter 1, Rules of the Road, presents a brief overview of the different ways research responsibilities are defined, ranging from formal regulations to informal codes and common practices.

Chapter 2, Research Misconduct, describes research practices that must be avoided and the obligation researchers have to report misconduct.

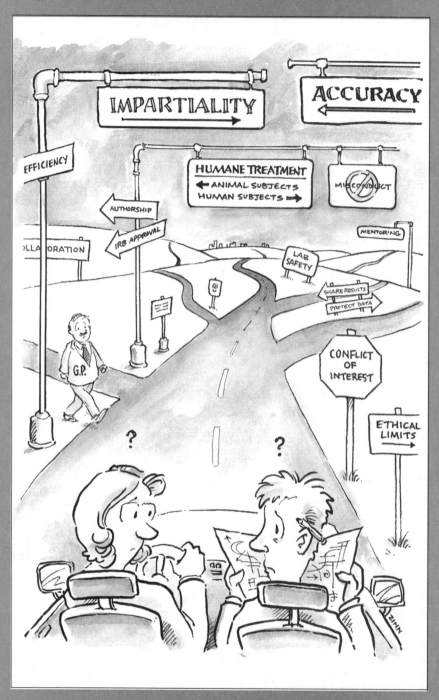

Setting off on the road to the responsible conduct of research

Chapter 1. Rules of the Road

How should you conduct your research? What practices should you follow? The public and their professional colleagues expect researchers to follow many rules and commonly accepted practices as they go about their work advancing knowledge and putting knowledge to work. Responsible conduct in research is conduct that meets this expectation.

Society's expectations for the responsible conduct of research are complex and not always well defined. Becoming a responsible researcher is not like becoming a responsible driver. Responsible driving is clearly defined through laws and written down in drivers' manuals. Before individuals are allowed to drive, they are tested on both their knowledge of the rules of the road and their skills. Then, licensed drivers are constantly reminded of their responsibilities by signs, traffic signals, and road markings. They also know that their behavior as drivers is monitored and that there are specific penalties for improper behavior.

Guidance for the responsible conduct of research is not this well organized. Some responsible practices are defined through law and institutional policies that *must be followed*. Others are set out in non-binding codes and guidelines that *should be followed*. Still other responsible practices are commonly accepted by most researchers but not written down. Instead, they are transmitted informally through mentoring, based on the understandings and values of each mentor. This situation is further complicated by the fact that researchers are not routinely tested on their knowledge of responsible practices or licensed. Moreover, their behavior as researchers is inconsistently monitored and the penalties for irresponsible behavior vary considerably.

Researchers do, of course, care deeply about responsible behavior in research and pay a great deal of attention to best research practices. The fact remains, however, that it can take some effort to find out what these practices are and how to act when the complex rules for responsible practice seem to conflict with one another.

This chapter describes the four basic sources of rules of the road for the responsible conduct of research:

✓ professional codes,

✓ government regulations,

✓ institutional policies, and

✓ personal convictions.

If you are primarily interested in learning more about your responsibilities rather than understanding their origin, skip ahead to the substantive chapters that follow, returning to this chapter later, when it might have more relevance.

Case Study

Katherine, a postdoc in Dr. Susan B.'s laboratory, has just had a manuscript accepted for publication in a prestigious research journal, conditional on a few important changes. Most importantly, the editor has requested that she significantly shorten the methods section to save space. If she makes the requested changes, other researchers may not be able to replicate her work.

Asked about the situation, Dr. B. recommends that Katherine go ahead with the changes. After all, if other researchers want more information they can always get in touch. She remains concerned that an inadequate explanation of her methods could lead other researchers to waste time and valuable research dollars attempting to replicate her work.

Should Katherine make the requested changes?

Should she be concerned about providing inadequate information to colleagues?

Is reducing detail in methods sections a reasonable way to go about saving valuable space in journals?

How can Katherine get definitive answers to these and other questions about the responsible conduct of research?

1a. Professional self-regulation

Prior to World War II, society provided little public support for research and did not expect much from researchers in return. Researchers were more or less left alone to run their own affairs, except when they assumed other roles, as teachers, physicians, or engineers.

As professionals, researchers have not been particularly concerned about rules for self-regulation. Since the goal of research is to advance knowledge through critical inquiry and scientific experimentation, it has commonly been assumed that the normal checking that goes on in testing new ideas is sufficient to keep researchers honest. Based on this assumption, research arguably does not need specific rules for self-regulation because it is, by definition, an activity that routinely monitors itself.

The lack of a perceived need for specific rules poses problems for researchers who want guidance on responsible research practices. Intellectually and professionally researchers organize their lives around fields of study. They are biologists, chemists, and physicists, increasingly working in specialized areas, such as biophysics, biochemistry, molecular biology, and so on. However, the societies that represent fields of study for the most part have not developed comprehensive guidelines for responsible research practices. Many do have codes of ethics, but most codes of ethics are simply general statements about ideals and do not contain the specific guidance researchers need to work responsibly in complex research settings.

Fortunately, there are a few important exceptions to this last generalization. Comprehensive descriptions of responsible research practices can be found in (see the resources listed at the end of this chapter for references):

National Academy of Sciences, On Being a Scientist (1995)

The scientific research enterprise, like other human activities, is built on a foundation of trust. Scientists trust that the results reported by others are valid. Society trusts that the results of research reflect an honest attempt by scientists to describe the world accurately and without bias. The level of trust that has characterized science and its relationship with society has contributed to a period of unparalleled scientific productivity. But this trust will endure only if the scientific community devotes itself to exemplifying and transmitting the values associated with ethical scientific conduct.

http://www.nap.edu/readingroom/books/obas/preface.html

✓ reports and policy statements issued by the National Academy of Sciences, the American Association for the Advancement of Science, the Association of American Medical Colleges, and Sigma Xi;

✓ guidance on responsible publication practices published in journals; and

✓ a few comprehensive professional codes.

When applicable, the guidance provided by professional societies is a good place to begin learning about responsible research practices.

American Chemical Society
The Chemist's Code of Conduct (1994)

Chemists Acknowledge Responsibilities To:

The Public.
: Chemists have a professional responsibly to serve the public interest and welfare and to further knowledge of science....

The Science of Chemistry.
: Chemists should seek to advance chemical science, understand the limitations of their knowledge, and respect the truth....

The Profession.
: Chemists should remain current with developments in their field, share ideas and information, keep accurate and complete laboratory records, maintain integrity in all conduct and publications, and give due credit to the contributions of others. Conflicts of interest and scientific misconduct, such as fabrication, falsification, and plagiarism, are incompatible with this Code.

The Employer.
: Chemists should promote and protect the legitimate interests of their employers, perform work honestly and competently, fulfill obligations, and safeguard proprietary information.

Employees.
: Chemists, as employers, should treat subordinates with respect for their professionalism and concern for their well-being....

Students.
: Chemists should regard the tutelage of students as a trust conferred by society for the promotion of the student's learning and professional development....

Associates.
: Chemists should treat associates with respect, regardless of the level of their formal education, encourage them, learn with them, share ideas honestly, and give credit for their contributions.

http://www.chemistry.org

1b. Government regulation

As public support for research grew after World War II, the public, through its elected officials, became more interested in the way research is practiced. Over time, concerns began to surface about some of these practices, focusing initially on the use of animals and humans in research and later on research misconduct. When it appeared that the research community was not doing enough to address these concerns, government turned to regulation.

Government regulations usually begin in Congress. When a potential problem is identified, Congress calls hearings to learn more about the problem and then passes legislation to fix it. The regulations covering the use of humans and animals in research as well as research misconduct stem from three acts passed by Congress:

✓   the 1966 Animal Welfare Act (PL 89-544),

✓   the 1974 National Research Act (PL 93-348), and

✓   the 1985 Health Research Extension Act (PL 99-158).

These and other research-related acts give the Federal Government the authority to regulate the research it funds.

Along with the authority to address problems, Congress usually provides guidance on general objectives, but it seldom drafts detailed regulations. This job falls to the Federal agencies in the Executive Branch of government, which are responsible for carrying out the law. Federal agencies translate Congressional directives into regulations (also called rules), policies, and guidelines.

In 1989, the Department of Health and Human Services (HHS) established the Office of Scientific Integrity (OSI) and the Office of Scientific Integrity Review (OSIR), in response to the 1985 Health Research Extension Act. The Office of Research Integrity (ORI) was established in 1992 and assumed the responsibilities previously assigned to

OSI and OSIR. In addition to responding to misconduct, ORI undertook a number of steps to promote integrity and responsible research practices. The *ORI Introduction to RCR* is a result of that effort.

Regulations. When Federal agencies translate Congressional directives into regulations, they must follow provisions set out in the Federal Administrative Procedure Act (5 USC 551-702). As its name implies, this act establishes procedures for developing new regulations, including steps for getting public input. Before establishing a new regulation, an agency must issue a draft regulation, obtain and consider public comment, and then issue the final regulation. Each step must be published in the *Federal Register*–the "official daily publication for rules, proposed rules, and notices of Federal agencies and organizations, as well as executive orders and other presidential documents" (http://www.gpoaccess.gov/fr/index.html). Objections raised during the public comment period must be addressed before the final regulation is adopted. After it is adopted, the final regulation is incorporated into the Code of Federal Regulations and becomes official government regulatory policy that must be followed.

Agency policies and guidelines. Executive Branch agencies have the authority to issue some policies as part of their normal operation. The National Institutes of Health (NIH), for example, has the authority to establish policies for grant awards. From time to time, it changes these policies to assure that its research funds are spent wisely and responsibly. It is in this capacity that NIH issued a special RCR "Training Grant Requirement" in 1989 and the more recent "Required Education in the Protection of Human Research Participants" (discussed in Chapter 3).

Federal agencies also issue Guidelines, which recommend but do not require a particular course of action. To help research institutions handle allegations of research

Required Education in the Protection of Human Research Participants
June 5, 2000 (Revised August 25, 2000)
National Institutes of Health

Policy: Beginning on October 1, 2000, the NIH will require education on the protection of human research participants for all investigators submitting NIH applications for grants or proposals for contracts or receiving new or non-competing awards for research involving human subjects.

Background: To bolster the Federal commitment to the protection of human research participants, several new initiatives to strengthen government oversight of medical research were announced by HHS Secretary Shalala on May 30, 2000. This announcement also reminds institutions of their responsibility to oversee their clinical investigators and institutional review boards (IRBs). One of the new initiatives addresses education and training. This NIH announcement is developed in response to the Secretary's directive.

http://grants2.nih.gov/grants/guide/notice-files/NOT-OD-00-039.html

misconduct (see Chapter 2), ORI issued as guidelines a Model Policy and Procedures for Responding to Allegations of Scientific Misconduct (http://ori.hhs.gov/policies/model_policy.shtml). In this case, the model policy is intended to provide guidance and does not impose binding requirements on institutions.

The plethora of Federal regulations, policies, and guidelines that affect research can be confusing. They do not always speak with one voice. The same aspect of a research project can be subject to regulations by more than one Federal agency, as for example the use of human or animal subjects. Common Federal regulations, such as the Federal Policy on Research Misconduct (discussed in Chapter 2) and the "Common Rule" for human subjects research (discussed in Chapter 3), are not truly common regulations until they have been adopted by all agencies. In addition, distinctions between regulations, policies, requirements, guidelines, and recommended practices can be difficult to understand.

Researchers are well advised to seek help when it comes to understanding Federal and state research regulations. The Federal agencies that regulate research have comprehensive Web pages that list and explain their policies and regulations and readily answer questions. For local advice, your institutional research administrators may be the best place to begin.

1c. Institutional policies

Research institutions (universities, hospitals, private research companies, and so on) are required by law to have policies that cover various aspects of their research programs if they accept Federal funds. They must have committees to review human and animal research (discussed in Chapters 3 and 4). They must have procedures for investigating and reporting research misconduct (Chapter 2) and conflicts of interest (Chapter 5). They must approve and manage all research budgets, ensure that laboratory safety rules are followed, and follow established practices for the responsible use of hazardous substances in research. They must also provide training for researchers who use animal or human subjects in their research and for individuals supported on NIH training grants.

To help manage their responsibilities, most research institutions have research offices/officers and institutional research policies. Both provide excellent sources of guidance for responsible conduct in research, since both are the products of the institution's efforts to clarify its own responsibilities. In addition, institutional policies are often more comprehensive than Federal and state policies since they must encompass the full panoply of institutional responsibilities. So, for example, many research institutions have more comprehensive definitions of research misconduct than the Federal Government to cover other practices that can undermine the integrity of research, such as the deliberate violation of research regulations, abuses of confidentiality, and even the failure to report misconduct (discussed in Chapter 2). Most also require institutional review for more human subjects research than is required by Federal regulation.

Large research institutions usually have Web sites that contain some or all of the following information:

✓ copies of institutional research policies,

✓ links to state and Federal policies,

✓ required forms and instructions for completing them,

✓ responsible conduct of research training programs, and

✓ lists of key personnel.

There is, of course, little or no coordination across different research institutions, so the information on an institution's Web site pertains only to that institution. But if you are looking for a comprehensive set of rules of the road for responsible research, check your home institution's research administration Web site or one from a comparable institution.

Stanford University - Research Policy Handbook
Document 2.1

Title:	Principles Concerning Research
Originally issued:	Dec 8, 1971
Current version:	Dec 8, 1971
Classification:	Stanford University Policy
Summary:	Presents broad principles to guide the research enterprise and assure the integrity of scholarly inquiry at Stanford University.

http://www.stanford.edu/dept/DoR/rph/2-1.html

1d. Personal responsibility

As important as rules of the road are for the responsible conduct of research, they have two important limitations. First, rules generally set minimum standards for behavior rather than strive for the ideal. The rules say that you can drive at 65 miles per hour over a stretch of road, but there may be times or circumstances when 55 would be better. If you use human subjects in research, you must follow specific rules, but there may be situations in which you should strive for a higher standard of conduct. Responsible research requires more than simply following rules.

Second, rules will not resolve some of the personal conflicts and moral dilemmas that arise in research. Journals have rules against listing undeserving authors on papers (individuals who have not made significant contributions to the research described in the paper). These same rules do not tell you what to do if the undeserving author can have a significant influence on your career. Rules also cannot replace the critical reasoning skills needed to assess ethically controversial human or animal experiments or conflicts of interest. Researchers will face ethical dilemmas in research. They should be able to recognize these dilemmas and know how to resolve them (discussed in Chapter 11).

The rules of the road for research therefore need to be supplemented with good judgment and a strong sense of personal integrity. When meeting deadlines, you can cut corners by filling in a few missing data points without actually running the experiments or adding a few references to your notes that you have not read. You can resist sharing data with colleagues or leave some information on method out of a publication to slow down the competition. You can ignore your responsibilities to students or a mentor in order to get your own work done. You can do all of these things and more, but should you?

In the final analysis, whatever decision you make when you confront a difficult decision about responsibility in research, you are the one who has to live with the consequences of that decision. If you are uncertain whether a particular course of action is responsible, subject it to one simple test. Imagine what you are preparing to do will be reported the next day on the front page of your local newspaper. If you are comfortable having colleagues, friends, and family know what you did, chances are you acted responsibly, provided, of course, you also understand your responsibilities as a researcher, as described in the rules of the road covered in the rest of the *ORI Introduction to RCR.*

Questions for discussion

1. **Is research a profession?**

2. **How do researchers learn about the responsible conduct of research?**

3. **How should researchers learn about the responsible conduct of research?**

4. **What factors influence researchers' attitudes toward the responsible conduct of research?**

5. **How is integrity in research monitored? Is self-regulation of integrity in research effective?**

Resources

Policies, Reports, and Policy Statements

Association of American Medical Colleges. *Developing a Code of Ethics in Research: A Guide for Scientific Societies*, Washington, DC: AAMC, 1997. (available at: https://services.aamc.org/Publications/index.cfm?fuseaction=Product.displayForm&prd_id=28&prv_id=17&cfid=1&cftoken=28C93522-2734-4BCC-92A8B871AE78AE22/)

Institute of Medicine. *The Responsible Conduct of Research in the Health Sciences*, Washington, DC: National Academies of Science, 1989. (available at: http://www.nap.edu/books/0309062373/html)

National Academy of Sciences. Committee on the Conduct of Science. *On Being a Scientist: Responsible Conduct in Research,* 2nd ed. Washington, DC: National Academy Press, 1995. (available at: http://www.nap.edu/readingroom/books/obas/)

National Institutes of Health. *Guidelines for the Conduct of Research in the Intramural Research Programs at NIH*, 1997. (available at: http://www.nih.gov/campus/irnews/guidelines.htm)

Sigma Xi. *Honor in Science*, New Haven, CN: Sigma Xi, 1984. (available at: http://www.sigmaxi.org/resources/publications/)

General Information Web Sites

American Association for the Advancement of Science. *Integrity in Scientific Research*. http://www.aaas.org/spp/video/ (Information on five videos on integrity in research.)

Bird, S, Spier, R, eds. *Science and Engineering Ethics*, 1995 ff. http://www.springer.com/east/home?SGWID=5-102-70-173705003-0&changeHeade/ (Includes articles on the responsible conduct of research.)

Collaborative Institutional Training Initiative (CITI), Course in the Responsible Conduct of Research. *Home Page.* https://www.citiprogram.org/rcrpage.asp?affiliation=100/

National Institutes of Health. *Research Conduct and Ethics Instruction Materials*. http://www1.od.nih.gov/oir/sourcebook/ResEthicsCases/cases-toc.htm

North Carolina State University. *Research & Professional Ethics Program*. http://www.fis.ncsu.edu/Grad/ethics/

Office of Research Integrity. *Home Page.* http://ori.hhs.gov/

Online Ethics Center for Engineering and Science. *Home Page.* http://onlineethics.org/

RCR Education Consortium. *Home Page.* http://rcrec.org/

Shamoo, AE, ed. *Accountability in Research: Policies and Quality Assurance*, 1994 ff. http://www.tandf.co.uk/journals/titles/08989621.html (Includes articles on research integrity and related issues.)

Additional Reading

Barnbaum, DR, Byron, M. *Research Ethics: Text and Readings*, Upper Saddle River, NJ: Prentice Hall, 2001.

Beach, D. *The Responsible Conduct of Research*, New York: VCH Publishers, 1996.

Bulger, RE, Heitman, E, Reiser, SJ. *The Ethical Dimensions of the Biological and Health Sciences*, 2nd ed. Cambridge, UK; New York: Cambridge University Press, 2002.

Elliott, D, Stern, JE. *Research Ethics: A Reader*, Hanover, NH: Published by University Press of New England for the Institute for the Study of Applied and Professional Ethics at Dartmouth College, 1997.

Frankel, M, Bird, S. eds. "The Role of Scientific Societies in Promoting Research Integrity," *Science and Engineering Ethics* 9, 2 (2003).

Grinnell, F. *The Scientific Attitude*, 2nd ed. New York: The Guilford Press, 1992.

Korenman, SG, Shipp, AC. *Teaching the Responsible Conduct of Research through a Case Study Approach: A Handbook for Instructors*, Washington, DC: Association of American Medical Colleges, 1994.

Macrina, FL. *Scientific Integrity: An Introductory Text with Cases*, 2nd ed. Washington, DC: ASM Press, 2000.

Penslar, RL. *Research Ethics: Cases and Materials*, Bloomington: Indiana University Press, 1995.

Resnik, DB. *The Ethics of Science : An Introduction, Philosophical Issues in Science*, London; New York: Routledge, 1998.

Shamoo, AE, Resnik, DB. *Responsible Conduct of Research*, New York: Oxford University Press, 2003.

Sigma Xi. *The Responsible Researcher: Paths and Pitfalls*, 1999.

Stern, JE, Elliott, D. *The Ethics of Scientific Research: A Guidebook for Course Development*, Hanover, NH: University Press of New England, 1997.

Whitbeck, C. *Ethics in Engineering Practice and Research*, Cambridge; New York: Cambridge University Press, 1998.

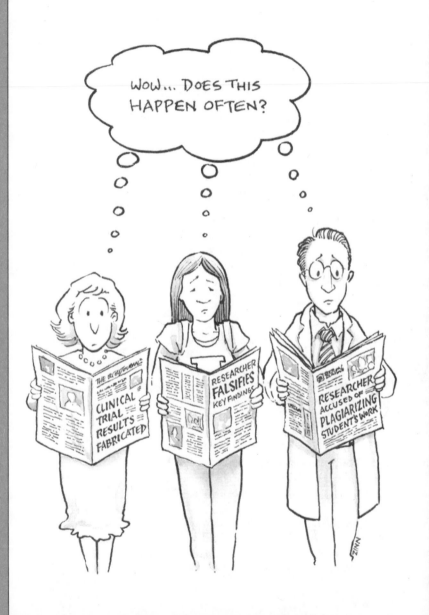

When research misconduct becomes public

Chapter 2. Research Misconduct

P ublic concern about misconduct in research first surfaced in the early 1980's following reports of cases of egregious misbehavior. One researcher republished under his own name dozens of articles previously published by others. Other researchers in one way or another falsified or fabricated research results. To make matters worse, it seemed as if research institutions sometimes ignored or deliberately covered up problems rather than investigate them. Eventually Congress stepped in and required Federal agencies and research institutions to develop research misconduct policies.

Research misconduct policies provide guidance on responsible conduct in three areas. They:

✓ establish definitions for misconduct in research,

✓ outline procedures for reporting and investigating misconduct, and

✓ provide protection for whistleblowers (persons who report misconduct) and persons accused of misconduct.

Together, the definitions of and procedures for handling allegations of misconduct in research form an initial foundation for effective self-regulation in research.

Although Federal policies technically apply only to federally funded research, many research institutions apply Federal research misconduct policies to all research. Many research institutions have also broadened the basic Federal definitions to include other inappropriate practices. In combination, Federal and institutional research misconduct policies define research practices that researchers must avoid. Failure to do so can result in the termination of employment or ineligibility to receive Federal funding.

Case Study

D r. José M. is beginning his fifth year as an independent researcher. His work is going well. He has published a number of important articles and secured a large grant for future work. Based on this progress, he expects his pending promotion review to proceed without problems.

Late one afternoon a graduate student hands José two papers written by a senior colleague in his department. She has circled graphs in each of the papers that are clearly the same but reported as representing two different experiments. After checking the graphs carefully and reviewing the supporting data, José agrees that something is wrong. The senior colleague, who will almost certainly be a member of his promotion review, has either made a careless mistake or falsified information in a publication. What should he do?

Ask the senior colleague about the graphs?

Bring the publications to the attention of his department chair?

Report the problem anonymously to a research administrator?

Encourage the graduate student to report the problem?

Nothing, at least until after the promotion review is completed?

2a. Federal research misconduct definition and policies

After a decade of sometimes spirited debate, in December 2000 the Office of Science and Technology Policy (OSTP) in the Executive Office of the President adopted a Federal Policy on Research Misconduct. The OSTP Policy is in most respects similar to earlier ones adopted by the Public Health Service (PHS) and the National Science Foundation (NSF), but it did recommend some significant changes to the definition of research misconduct. When it is finally implemented by all government research agencies (the target date of December 2001 was not met), all federally funded researchers will be subject to a uniform definition of research misconduct.

Definition. The OSTP Policy defines "research misconduct" as "fabrication, falsification, or plagiarism in proposing, performing, or reviewing research, or in reporting research results" (see accompanying box for details). It also sets the legal threshold for proving charges of misconduct.

To be considered research misconduct, actions must:

✓ represent a "significant departure from accepted practices";

✓ have been "committed intentionally, or knowingly, or recklessly"; and

✓ be "proven by a preponderance of evidence."

These further stipulations limit the Federal Government's role in research misconduct (fabrication, falsification, or plagiarism) to well-documented, serious departures from accepted research practices.

When using the common Federal definition to discuss research misconduct, it is important to understand that it establishes a minimum standard for measuring acceptable behavior, not a standard for judging all research behavior. In particular, it does not imply that all other behaviors are acceptable. It also does not encompass criminal behavior, personal disputes, violations of grant management policies or other unacceptable behaviors not unique to research, such as discrimination or harrassment. The government's main concern in establishing this definition is to assure that publicly funded research is accurate and appropriately represented by clearly stating that three practices, commonly referred to as "FFP," are wrong.

Federal Research Misconduct Policy.

I. Research Misconduct Defined. Research misconduct is defined as fabrication, falsification, or plagiarism in proposing, performing, or reviewing research, or in reporting research results.

- Fabrication is making up data or results and recording or reporting them.

- Falsification is manipulating research materials, equipment, or processes, or changing or omitting data or results such that the research is not accurately represented in the research record.

- Plagiarism is the appropriation of another person's ideas, processes, results, or words without giving appropriate credit.

- Research misconduct does not include differences of opinion.

http://ori.hhs.gov/policies/fed_research_misconduct.shtml

Reporting and investigation. Federal misconduct policy assumes that researchers and research institutions bear the primary responsibility for reporting and investigating allegations of misconduct. This assumption is consistent with the position, strongly supported by most researchers, that research is a profession and should regulate its own conduct (see Chapter 1).

Successful professional self-regulation depends on conscientious community participation. For individual researchers, this means they must assume responsibility for their own actions, take misconduct seriously, and report apparent misconduct by other researchers.

Every institution that receives PHS funding must have procedures in place for receiving and investigating reports of research misconduct. These procedures must include:

✓ the designation of individuals who are authorized to receive and investigate allegations of misconduct,

✓ provisions for an initial inquiry to determine whether the allegations have any merit,

✓ provisions for a formal investigation to reach conclusions about the truth of the allegations,

✓ the designation of an individual who is authorized to weigh (adjudicate) the conclusions reached in the investigation and impose administrative actions to redress the misconduct (sanctions) or take steps to vindicate the person charged, and

✓ provisions for reporting findings to ORI.

Researchers should be familiar with these procedures and their institution's definition of research misconduct (discussed below).

Basic protections. Researchers who commit misconduct place their careers at risk. The Federal Government can debar researchers who commit misconduct from receiving Federal funds for a specified period of time. In most instances, research institutions also take their own actions, such as terminating a researcher's employment or requiring supervision of future research activities. By like token, making allegations of misconduct—blowing the whistle— can sometimes place a whistleblower's career at risk. Although by law institutions must not retaliate against whistleblowers who report in good faith, they sometimes do.

The new common Federal policy provides guidelines for protecting both parties—the whistleblower and the respondent—in research misconduct investigations. As a general rule, research misconduct allegations must not be made public until they have been fully investigated and confirmed. There are, however, exceptions to this rule. If the misconduct could pose a threat to public health or safety, such as misconduct in a clinical trial, it must immediately be brought to the attention of the person heading the trial, the person with oversight authority, or both. ORI and the Federal sponsor must also be notified immediately. In such cases, the names of the persons charged should remain confidential, but steps must be taken to safeguard the subjects in the trial.

Similarly, research institutions and researchers must not in any way penalize or take action against individuals who report research misconduct in good faith. Even if accusations are not sustained, as long as they are brought in good faith, informants must be protected and given support since they play a vital role in professional self-regulation.

2b. Institutional research misconduct policies

Institutional research misconduct policies generally follow the pattern recommended by the Federal Government, but almost always include some additional elements that for one reason or another are assumed to have local importance. This is particularly true for the definition of research misconduct. Institutional definitions must include some

University Research Misconduct Policies

Rice University. Research misconduct may include the fabrication/ falsification of data, plagiarism, or other practices that seriously deviate from those that are commonly accepted within the scientific community for proposing, conducting, reviewing, or reporting research. It also encompasses the failure to comply with federal requirements for protecting researchers, human and animal subjects, and the public. In general, gross negligence of research standards and any action taken with the intent to defraud are considered forms of research misconduct. It does not, however, include honest error or honest differences in interpreting or judging data.

http://professor.rice.edu/professor/Research_Misconduct.asp

University of New Mexico. A researcher commits research misconduct under UNM's policy if he or she fabricates or falsifies data or research results or plagiarizes another person's ideas or work. Research misconduct also occurs if a researcher wantonly disregards truth or objectivity or fails to comply or attempt to comply with legal requirements governing the research; however, other University policies and procedures will be followed in resolving such cases. It is important to understand that research misconduct is not a mistake in reasoning, disagreeing with recognized authorities, misinterpreting results, an error in planning or carrying out an experiment, or an oversight in attribution.

http://www.unm.edu/%7Ecounsel/research/policies/2464.pdf

version of FFP, but then sometimes add other practices that also constitute misconduct in the particular local setting. Thus, depending on where a researcher works, any of the following practices could be reported as misconduct in research.

Violation of Federal rules. As will be discussed in later chapters, research is subject to many rules or regulations other than research misconduct policies. Although the violation of a research rule or regulation is not considered misconduct under the common Federal definition of research misconduct, many research institutions explicitly state that the violation of any research regulation is research misconduct.

Abuse of confidentiality. Confidentiality plays a number of important roles in research. Most peer review is done confidentially (see Chapter 10). Researchers also share ideas with colleagues with the understanding that they will not be used or made public without permission (see Chapter 8). Federal regulations, such as the Health Insurance Portability and Accountability Act of 1996 (see Chapter 3), impose confidentiality requirements on human subjects research. The abuse of confidentiality may not undermine the validity of research data, but it can undermine the integrity of the research process. Therefore, some institutions include such abuses under their definition of research misconduct.

Authorship and publication violations. As will be discussed in Chapter 9, there are well-established guidelines for getting credit for work done (authorship) and making research results known (publication). Some violations of these guidelines do not rise to the level of FFP, as defined in Federal policy. For example, the Federal Government usually does not get involved in disputes over authorship or investigate charges of trivial publication (dividing the results of a single experiment into multiple publications so that there are more to list on a résumé). However, given the importance of the integrity of the research record, some research institutions include authorship and publication violations in their misconduct policies.

Failure to report misconduct. Failure to report many crimes can be considered a crime and result in penalties. This is particularly true if failure to report a crime puts other individuals or society at risk. Research misconduct can put individuals at risk, if, for example, the misconduct affects information that is used for making medical or public decisions. Failure to report research misconduct also undermines professional self-regulation. Therefore, some research institutions include failure to report misconduct in their research misconduct policies.

Obstruction of investigations and retaliation. To emphasize the importance of research misconduct investigations, some institutions also include obstruction of investigations and retaliation against whistleblowers under research misconduct.

Other practices. Early in the evolution of Federal research misconduct policies, the National Science Foundation (NSF) and the Public Health Service (PHS) included a broad provision in their definitions to catch other practices that "seriously deviate" from commonly accepted practices. NSF in particular felt that FFP left out behaviors that could undermine the integrity of the research it funded. While the "serious deviations" clause no longer exists in the common Federal definition, except as a standard for judging FFP, it can still be found in some institutional policies. Researchers therefore need to be aware of the fact that in some settings, actions that seriously deviate from commonly accepted practices can be considered research misconduct.

2c. Putting research misconduct into perspective

Research misconduct has understandably received considerable public attention. Researchers who act dishonestly waste public funds, harm the research record, distort the research process, undermine public trust, and can even adversely impact public health and safety. Research misconduct policies, whether Federal, state, institutional, or professional, identify seriously inappropriate behaviors and establish procedures for dealing with them.

Judged on the basis of the number of confirmed cases, misconduct apparently is not common in research. Over the last decade, PHS and NSF combined have averaged no more than 20 to 30 misconduct findings a year. This puts the annual rate of misconduct in research at or below 1 case for every 10,000 researchers. However, before making too much of this assessment, two important cautions need to be kept in mind.

First, the number of confirmed cases is probably less than the number of actual cases. Underreporting is to be expected, as it is in criminal and other types of inappropriate behavior. Moreover, several studies have suggested that researchers do not report suspected misconduct, even though they should (see Korenman, Additional Reading). Since every case of misconduct can potentially undermine public support for research, researchers should take their responsibility to look out for and report research misconduct seriously.

Second, the responsibility to avoid misconduct in research is a minimum standard for the responsible conduct of research, so the fact that most researchers do not engage in research misconduct does not necessarily imply that the level of integrity in research overall is high. Responsible research requires careful attention to many other expectations for appropriate practice, as discussed in the remainder of the *ORI Introduction to RCR*.

Questions for discussion

1. Should other practices besides fabrication, falsification, and plagiarism be considered misconduct in research?

2. Is it fair to use "significant departure from accepted practices" to make judgments about a researcher's behavior?

3. Should researchers report misconduct if they are concerned that doing so could adversely impact their career?

4. What evidence is needed to demonstrate that a researcher committed misconduct "intentionally, or knowingly, or recklessly"?

5. What are appropriate penalties for different types of misconduct?

Resources

Policies, Reports, and Policy Statements

Department of Health and Human Services. Commission on Research Integrity. *Integrity and Misconduct in Research*, Washington, DC: Health and Human Services, 1995. (available at: http://ori.hhs. gov/documents/report_commission.pdf)

Department of Health and Human Services. *Public Health Service Policies on Research Misconduct; Final Rule,* 42 CFR Parts 50 and 93, (2005). (available at: http://ori.hhs.gov/policies/federal_policies. shtml)

National Academy of Science. Committee on Science Engineering and Public Policy. Panel on Scientific Responsibility and the Conduct of Research. *Responsible Science*: *Ensuring the Integrity of the Research Process*, Washington, DC: National Academy Press, 1992.

Office of the President. Office of Science and Technology Policy. "Federal Policy on Research Misconduct," *Federal Register* 65 (6 December 2000): 76260-64. (available at: http://ori.hhs.gov/ policies/fed_research_misconduct.shtml)

Office of Research Integrity, *ORI Model Policy and Procedures for Responding to Allegations of Scientific Misconduct*, 1995, revised 1997. (available at: http://ori.hhs.gov/policies/model_policy.shtml)

National Science Foundation. *Research Misconduct*, 45 CFR 689 (2002). (available at: http://www.nsf.gov/oig/misconscieng.jsp)

United States. Congress. House. Committee on Science and Technology. Subcommittee on Investigations and Oversight. *Fraud in Biomedical Research*, Washington, DC: GPO, 1981.

Wells, FO, Lock, S, Farthing, MJG. *Fraud and Misconduct in Biomedical Research*, London: BMJ Books, 2001.

General Information Web Sites

National Science Foundation, Office of Inspector General. *Home Page*. http://www.oig.nsf.gov/

Office of Research Integrity. *Handling Misconduct*. http://ori.hhs. gov/misconduct/

Additional Reading

Braxton, JM, Bayer, AE. "Perceptions of Research Misconduct and an Analysis of their Correlates." In *Perspectives on Scholarly Misconduct in the Sciences*, edited by John M. Braxton, Columbus, OH: Ohio State University Press, 1999, 236-258.

Korenman, SG, Berk, R, Wenger, NS, Lew, V. "Evaluation of the Research Norms of Scientists and Administrators Responsible for Academic Research Integrity," *Journal of the American Medical Association* 279, 1 (1998): 41-47.

Parrish, DM. "Scientific Misconduct and Correcting the Scientific Literature," *Academic Medicine* 74, 3 (1999): 221-230.

Pascal, CB. "Scientific Misconduct and Research Integrity for the Bench Scientist," *Proceedings of the Society for Experimental Biology and Medicine* 224, 4 (2000): 220-230.

Price, AR. "Anonymity and Pseudonymity in Whistleblowing to the U.S. Office of Research Integrity," *Academic Medicine* 73, 5 (1998): 467-472.

Rhoades, LR. "The American Experience: Lessons Learned," *Science and Engineering Ethics* 6,1 (2000): 95-107.

School of Education. University of Indiana. *Understanding Plagiarism*, 2002. (available at: http://education.indiana. edu/~frick/plagiarism)

United States. President's Commission for the Study of Ethical Problems in Medicine and Biomedical and Behavioral Research. *Whistleblowing in Biomedical Research: Policies and Procedures for Responding to Reports of Misconduct: Proceedings of a Workshop, September 21-22, 1981*, Washington, DC: GPO, 1981.

Part II.

Planning Research

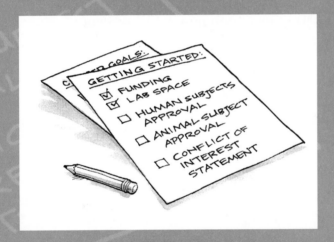

Part II: Planning Research

RESEARCH BEGINS WITH IDEAS, QUESTIONS

and hypotheses. What causes this

particular phenomenon? What would

happen if...? How can I find out...?

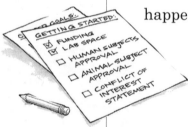

Researchers think first

about problems and ways

to solve them and about the resources

they will need to perform experiments.

P lanning for any project should include the consideration of responsibilities. In some cases, work cannot begin until it has been approved. In other cases, confronting potential problems before they arise can help ensure that they do not turn into real problems later.

The chapters in this section cover three areas where appropriate planning and approval are essential:

Chapter 3, The Protection of Human Subjects, describes the regulations covering the use of humans in research.

Chapter 4, The Welfare of Laboratory Animals, describes similar regulations for animals used in research.

Chapter 5, Conflicts of Interest, discusses what research-ers should do when their interests are or appear to be in conflict.

Planning is essential in other areas as well. Responsible research administration, the safe use of hazardous materials, and the fair treatment of students and employees should be addressed early in any project. However, with the use of humans and animals and, increasingly, the potential influence of conflicting interests, there is no choice. These responsibilities must be fully addressed before the first subject is contacted, the first animal purchased, or any agreement signed.

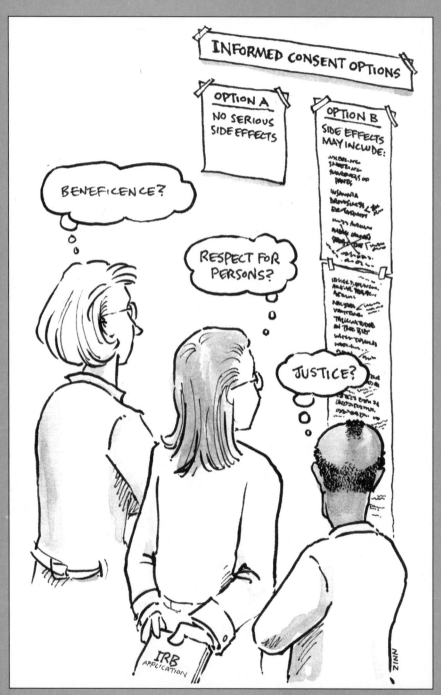

Designing a responsible informed consent form

Chapter 3. The Protection of Human Subjects

The use of human subjects in research benefits society in many ways, from contributing to the development of new drugs and medical procedures to understanding how we think and act. It also can and has imposed unacceptable risks on research subjects. To help ensure that the risks do not outweigh the benefits, human subjects research is carefully regulated by society.

Case Study

Two weeks into the new semester, the professor in Mary's course on family health gives the class a special assignment that was not on the course syllabus. Over the next week, everyone in the class is to talk with three classmates who are not in the course about the way their families deal with medical emergencies and chronic illness. Next week they should come to class prepared to report on their interviews. The Professor warns them, however, that in talking about their conversations they should not mention any names to protect the privacy of their classmates.

The assignment makes Mary uneasy. In her basic psychology course last semester she learned about some of the rules pertaining to the use of human subjects in research. However, when she raises her concerns with her professor, he assures her that her informal conversations with classmates are not research and therefore not subject to regulation. Moreover, since she will not be mentioning any names, there are no privacy issues to worry about.

> Should Mary be content with these assurances and conduct the interviews?
> If she still has concerns, where should she turn for advice?
> Did the professor act properly in giving this assignment to the class?

Investigators who conduct research involving humans that is subject to regulation must comply with all relevant Federal regulations as well as any applicable state and local laws, regulations, and policies related to the protection of human subjects. They are also expected to follow other relevant codes that have been formulated by professional groups. To meet these responsibilities requires, among other things:

✓ knowing what research is subject to regulation,

✓ understanding and following the rules for project approval,

✓ getting appropriate training, and

✓ accepting continuing responsibility for compliance through all stages of a project.

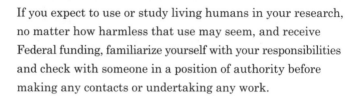 If you expect to use or study living humans in your research, no matter how harmless that use may seem, and receive Federal funding, familiarize yourself with your responsibilities and check with someone in a position of authority before making any contacts or undertaking any work.

3a. Federal regulations

Society protects the welfare of individuals in many ways, but it did not specifically address the issue of the welfare of research subjects until after World War II. Following the War, widespread concerns about atrocities committed during the War in the name of research led to the formulation of a code for human subjects research known as the Nuremberg Code (1947). Although not binding on researchers, the Nuremberg Code and the later Declaration of Helsinki (1964; latest revision and clarification, 2002) provided the first explicit international guidelines for the ethical treatment of human subjects in research.

The Nuremberg Code and Declaration of Helsinki did not put an end to unethical human subjects research. During the Cold War, U.S. researchers tested the effects of radiation on hospital patients, children, and soldiers without obtaining informed consent or permission to do so. Through the 1950's and 1960's, well after antibiotics effective for the treatment of syphilis were discovered, scores of African-American males in a long-term syphilis study (conducted by the U.S. Public Health Service in Tuskegee, Alabama) were not offered treatment with the new drugs so that researchers could continue to track the course of the disease. These and other questionable practices raised serious public concern and led eventually to government regulation.

Excerpts, Nuremberg Code (1947)

1. The voluntary consent of the human subject is absolutely essential.

2. The experiment should be such as to yield fruitful results for the good of society.

3. The experiment should be so designed and based on the results of animal experimentation and a knowledge of the natural history of the disease.

4. The experiment should be so conducted as to avoid all unnecessary physical and mental suffering and injury.

5. No experiment should be conducted where there is an a priori reason to believe that death or disabling injury will occur.

6. The degree of risk to be taken should never exceed that determined by the humanitarian importance of the problem to be solved by the experiment.

7. Proper preparations should be made and adequate facilities provided to protect the experimental subject against even remote possibilities of injury, disability, or death.

8. The experiment should be conducted only by scientifically qualified persons.

9. During the course of the experiment the human subject should be at liberty to bring the experiment to an end.

10. During the course of the experiment the scientist in charge must be prepared to terminate the experiment at any stage, if he has probable cause to believe, in the exercise of the good faith, superior skill and careful judgment required of him that a continuation of the experiment is likely to result in injury, disability, or death to the experimental subject.

http://www.hhs.gov/ohrp/references/nurcode.htm

To prevent these and similar abuses from continuing, in 1974 Congress required the Department of Health, Education and Welfare (HEW, currently Health and Human Services—HHS) to clarify its rules for the use of human subjects in research. With this mandate in hand, HEW codified its procedures under Title 45 of the Code of Federal Regulations, Part 46 (45 CFR 46). (At roughly the same time, the FDA codified its rules for human subjects research under 21 CFR 50 and 56.)

Congress also called in 1974 for the creation of a National Commission for the Protection of Human Subjects of

Biomedical and Behavioral Research. During the 4 years it met, the Commission issued a number of reports on the protection of research subjects and recommended principles for judging the ethics of human subjects research (discussed below).

In 1991 most Federal departments and agencies that conduct or support human subjects research adopted a common set of regulations for the protection of human subjects referred to as the "Common Rule" (45 CFR 46, Subpart A). Additional requirements on three sensitive research areas are also included in 45 CFR 46:

✓ Subpart B – Additional Protections for Pregnant Women, Human Fetuses and Neonates Involved in Research.

✓ Subpart C – Additional Protections Pertaining to Biomedical and Behavioral Research Involving Prisoners as Subjects.

✓ Subpart D – Additional Protections for Children Involved as Subjects in Research.

Together, 45 CFR 46, Subparts A-D, provide a comprehensive articulation of society's expectations for the responsible use of human subjects in research.

Authority for enforcing the HHS regulations for the protection of human subjects who participate in research conducted or supported by HHS now rests with the Office for Human Research Protections (OHRP) in the Office of Public Health and Science (OPHS). If you have specific questions about the Federal requirements for the protection of human subjects, contact your local institutional officials, OHRP (for research conducted or supported by HHS), or appropriate officials at the department or agency conducting or supporting the research.

3b. Definitions

Researchers are responsible for obtaining appropriate approval before conducting research involving human subjects. The need for approval rests on three seemingly obvious but not always easy-to-interpret considerations: 1) whether the work qualifies as research, 2) whether it involves human subjects, and 3) whether it is exempt. All three considerations are discussed in the Common Rule and guide decisionmaking about the use of human subjects in research. The authority to make decisions about the need for approval rests with the Institutional Review Board (IRB, discussed below) or other appropriate institutional officials.

Research. The Common Rule defines research as "systematic investigation, including research development, testing and evaluation, designed to develop or contribute to generalizable knowledge" (§ 46.102(d), see box, next page, for full definition). This means that a project or study is research if it:

✓ is conducted with the intention of drawing conclusions that have some general applicability and

✓ uses a commonly accepted scientific method.

The random collection of information about individuals that has no general applicability is not research. Scientific investigation that leads to generalizable knowledge is.

Human subjects. Human subjects are "living individual(s) about whom an investigator conducting research obtains: (1) data through intervention or interaction with the individual; or (2) identifiable private information" (§ 46.102(f), see box, next page, for full definition). Humans are considered subjects and covered by Federal regulations if the researcher:

✓ interacts or intervenes directly with them, or

✓ collects identifiable private information.

45 CFR 46. 102
Protection of Human Subjects – Definitions

(d) **Research** means a systematic investigation, including research development, testing and evaluation, designed to develop or contribute to generalizable knowledge. Activities which meet this definition constitute research for purposes of this policy, whether or not they are conducted or supported under a program which is considered research for other purposes. For example, some demonstration and service programs may include research activities.

- - - - - - - - - - - - - - -

(f) **Human subject** means a living individual about whom an investigator (whether professional or student) conducting research obtains

(1) data through intervention or interaction with the individual, or

(2) identifiable private information.

Intervention includes both physical procedures by which data are gathered (for example, venipuncture) and manipulations of the subject or the subject's environment that are performed for research purposes. Interaction includes communication or interpersonal contact between investigator and subject. Private information includes information about behavior that occurs in a context in which an individual can reasonably expect that no observation or recording is taking place, and information which has been provided for specific purposes by an individual and which the individual can reasonably expect will not be made public (for example, a medical record). Private information must be individually identifiable (i.e., the identity of the subject is or may readily be ascertained by the investigator or associated with the information) in order for obtaining the information to constitute research involving human subjects.

http://www.hhs.gov/ohrp/humansubjects/guidance/45cfr46.htm

If one of these two conditions applies and if the project or study qualifies as research, then institutional approval is needed before any work is undertaken.

Exempt research. Some studies that involve humans may be exempt from the requirements in the Federal regulations. Studies that fall into the following categories could qualify for exemptions, including:

✓ research conducted in established or commonly accepted educational settings;

✓ research involving the use of educational tests;

✓ research involving the collection or study of existing data, documents, records, pathological specimens, or diagnostic specimens, if unidentifiable or publicly available;

✓ research and demonstration projects which are conducted by or subject to the approval of department or agency heads; or

✓ taste and food quality evaluation and consumer acceptance studies.

It is critically important to note, however, that decisions about whether studies are exempt from the requirements of the Common Rule must be made by an IRB or an appropriate institutional official and not by the investigator.

3c. IRB membership and deliberations

Federally funded research that uses human subjects must be reviewed and approved by an independent committee called an Institutional Review Board or IRB. The IRB provides an opportunity and place for individuals with different backgrounds to discuss and make judgments about the acceptability of projects, based on criteria set out in the Common Rule.

Under the Common Rule, IRBs must have at least five members and include at least one scientist, one non-scientist, and "one member who is not otherwise affiliated with the institution and who is not part of the immediate family of a person who is affiliated with the institution" (§ 46.107(d)). IRBs have authority to approve, require modification of (in order to secure approval), and disapprove all research activities covered by the Common Rule. They also are responsible for conducting continuing review of research at least once per year and for ensuring that proposed changes in approved research are not initiated without IRB review and approval, except when necessary to eliminate apparent immediate hazards to the subject.

IRBs weigh many factors before approving proposals. Their main concern is to determine whether (§ 46.111(a)):

✓ risks to subjects are minimized;

✓ risks to subjects are reasonable in relation to anticipated benefits, if any, to subjects, and the importance of the knowledge that may reasonably be expected to result;

✓ selection of subjects is equitable;

✓ informed consent will be sought from each prospective subject or the subject's legally authorized representative;

✓ informed consent will be appropriately documented;

✓ when appropriate, the research plan makes adequate provision for monitoring the data collected to ensure the safety of subjects; and

✓ when appropriate, there are adequate provisions to protect the privacy of subjects and to maintain the confidentiality of data.

Researchers should consider each of these issues before completing their research plan and submitting it to an IRB for approval.

Making decisions about whether human subjects will be treated fairly and appropriately or given adequate information requires judgments about right and wrong (moral judgments). In the 1979 Belmont Report, the National Commission recommended three principles for making these judgments:

✓ **respect for persons** and their right to make decisions for and about themselves without undue influence or coercion from someone else (the researcher in most cases);

✓ **beneficence** or the obligation to maximize benefits and reduce risks to the subject; and

> ## The Belmont Report (1979)
> ### *Ethical Principles and Guidelines for the Protection of Human Subjects of Research*
>
> SUMMARY: On July 12, 1974, the National Research Act (Pub. L. 93-348) was signed into law, thereby creating the National Commission for the Protection of Human Subjects of Biomedical and Behavioral Research. One of the charges to the Commission was to identify the basic ethical principles that should underlie the conduct of biomedical and behavioral research involving human subjects and to develop guidelines which should be followed to assure that such research is conducted in accordance with those principles.
>
> http://www.hhs.gov/ohrp/humansubjects/guidance/belmont.htm

✓ **justice** or the obligation to distribute benefits and risks equally without prejudice to particular individuals or groups, such as the mentally disadvantaged or members of a particular race or gender.

While this list does not exhaust the principles that can be used for judging the ethics of human subjects research, it has nonetheless been accepted as a common standard for most IRB deliberations. Knowing this, researchers should spend time considering whether their work does provide adequate respect for persons, appropriately balances risks and benefits, and is just.

3d. Training

To help assure that researchers understand their responsibilities to research subjects, the National Institutes of Health (NIH) currently requires

…education on the protection of human research participants for all investigators submitting NIH applications for grants or proposals for contracts or receiving new or non-competing awards for research involving human subjects. (http://grants2.nih.gov/grants/guide/notice-files/NOT-OD-00-039.html)

Many institutions, including NIH, provide this training through special Web-based programs that summarize essential information and in some cases require some evidence of mastery. A description of the education program and who was trained must be included in applications for grants and contracts before they will be considered.

3e. Continuing responsibility

Once a project has been approved by an IRB, researchers must adhere to the approved protocol and follow any additional IRB instructions. This, unfortunately, is where a few researchers and institutions have occasionally run into problems and temporarily had their "assurance" (FWA - Federalwide Assurance) suspended. The continuing responsibilities that researchers have include:

✓ enrolling only those subjects that meet IRB approved inclusion and exclusion criteria,

Federalwide Assurance (FWA)

The Federal Policy (Common Rule) for the protection of human subjects at Section 103(a) requires that each institution "engaged" in Federally supported human subject research file an "Assurance" of protection for human subjects. The Assurance formalizes the institution's commitment to protect human subjects. The requirement to file an Assurance includes both "awardee" and collaborating "performance site" institutions.

Under the Federal Policy (Common Rule) at Section 102(f) awardees and their collaborating institutions become "engaged" in human subject research whenever their employees or agents (i) intervene or interact with living individuals for research purposes; or (ii) obtain, release, or access individually identifiable private information for research purposes.

In addition, awardee institutions are automatically considered to be "engaged" in human subject research whenever they receive a direct HHS award to support such research, even where all activities involving human subjects are carried out by a subcontractor or collaborator. In such cases, the awardee institution bears ultimate responsibility for protecting human subjects under the award. The awardee is also responsible for ensuring that all collaborating institutions engaged in the research hold an OHRP approved Assurance prior to their initiation of the research.

http://www.hhs.gov/ohrp/assurances/assurances_index.html

✓ properly obtaining and documenting informed consent,

✓ obtaining prior approval for any deviation from the approved protocol,

✓ keeping accurate records, and

✓ promptly reporting to the IRB any unanticipated problems involving risks to subjects or others.

While research institutions are increasingly monitoring the progress of human subjects research, the primary responsibility for conducting experiments as approved still lies with the individual researchers and staff who conduct the experiments.

3f. Ethical issues

Despite the many rules governing research with humans, tough choices continually arise that have no easy answers.

Informed consent. It is widely agreed that research subjects should be fully informed about experiments in which they may participate and give their consent before they enroll. However, some subjects, such as children, some adults with impaired decisionmaking capacity, and some critically ill patients, cannot give informed consent, either because they are not old enough to understand the information being conveyed or because they have lost their ability to understand.

These and other problems could be eliminated by forbidding researchers to do studies that raise difficult questions about respect for persons, beneficence, and justice, but this would make it difficult or even impossible to get some crucial information needed to make informed decisions about medicine and public health. Since children do not respond to medicines in the same way as adults, it is important to include children in some clinical trials. However, it is not easy to decide when they should be included and how consent can/should be obtained.

Right to withdraw. It is widely agreed that research subjects should have the right to withdraw from experiments at any time, but in some cases they cannot. In the final stages of development, mechanical hearts are tested on patients whose own heart is about to fail. But if it has not failed, and once the mechanical heart replaces the weakened heart, there is no turning back. The patient can technically withdraw from the experiment and undergo no further testing, but he or she cannot withdraw from the conditions imposed by the experiment, no matter how distressing living with the mechanical heart might be. Knowing this, under what conditions should these experiments be allowed?

Risk without benefit. In one recent experiment, researchers wanted to test whether a common surgical procedure used to relieve arthritis pain had any benefits. To gather information about benefits they designed a clinical trial in which subjects in the control group received sham surgery. An operation was performed, but the common surgical procedure was not performed.

The researchers in this case complied with all regulations, which included thorough IRB review. None of the patients experienced any adverse effects, and the study concluded that the common surgical procedure did not provide significant benefits. However, since surgery always involves some risk, the subjects in the control group were placed at risk without any expectation that they would benefit. Should this be allowed, and if so, under what circumstances?

These and other questions must ultimately be answered by IRBs during the review process. Researchers who serve on IRBs need additional training to help them deal with the growing complexities of biomedical, social, and behavioral research. Researchers who use human subjects in research should seriously consider having some formal training in bioethics so that they can participate in the critical reasoning process needed to respond to the complex moral issues raised by the use of human subjects in research.

Questions for discussion

1. Why should some research on humans be exempted from regulation?

2. What other criteria could be used to identify necessary members for IRBs?

3. What should subjects know about proposed research and their protection before they enroll as subjects?

4. What other principles could be used for evaluating the ethics of human subjects research besides respect for persons, beneficence, and justice?

5. Should subjects be allowed to enroll in experiments that either promise no direct benefit to them or cannot provide them with the opportunity to withdraw completely?

Resources

Policies, Reports, and Policy Statements

Directives for Human Experimentation: Nuremberg Code. 1949. (available at: http://www.hhs.gov/ohrp/references/nurcode.htm)

Federal Policy for the Protection of Human Subjects, 45 CFR 46, Subpart A (2005). (available at: http://www.hhs.gov/ohrp/humansubjects/guidance/45cfr46.htm)

National Institutes of Health. *Guidelines for the Conduct of Research Involving Human Subjects at the National Institutes of Health*, 1995. (available at: http://www.nihtraining.com/ohsrsite/guidelines/graybook.html)

———. *Required Education in the Protection of Human Research Participants*, National Institutes of Health, 2000. (available at: http://grants2.nih.gov/grants/guide/notice-files/NOT-OD-00-039.html)

The National Commission for the Protection of Human Subjects of Biomedical and Behavioral Research. *The Belmont Report: Ethical Principles and Guidelines for the Protection of Human Subjects of Research*, Washington, DC: DHHS, 1979. (available at: http://www.hhs.gov/ohrp/humansubjects/guidance/belmont.htm)

World Medical Association. *Declaration of Helsinki: Ethical Principles for Medical Research Involving Human Subjects*, Helsinki, Finland: World Medical Association, 1964, 2002. (available at: http://www.wma.net/e/policy/b3.htm)

General Information Web Sites

Food and Drug Administration. *Information Sheet: Guidance for Institutional Review Boards and Clinical Investigators*, 1998. http://www.fda.gov/oc/ohrt/irbs/default.htm

National Institutes of Health. *Standards for Clinical Research within the NIH Intramural Research Program*, 2000. http://www.cc.nih.gov/ccc/clinicalresearch/index.html

National Institutes of Health. *Bioethics Resources on the Web*, 2003. http://bioethics.od.nih.gov/

———. *OHSR Infosheets/Forms*, nd. http://ohsr.od.nih.gov/info/info.html

National Institutes of Health, Office of Human Subjects Research. *Home Page*. http://ohsr.od.nih.gov/index.html

Office for Human Research Protections, HHS. *Home Page*. http://www.hhs.gov/ohrp/

Additional Reading

Eckstein, S, King's College (University of London). Centre of Medical Law and Ethics. *Manual for Research Ethics Committees*, 6th ed. Cambridge, UK; New York: Cambridge University Press, 2003.

Federman, DD, Hanna, KE, Rodriguez, LL. Institute of Medicine (U.S.). Committee on Assessing the System for Protecting Human Research Participants. *Responsible Research: A Systems Approach to Protecting Research Participants*, Washington, D.C.: National Academies Press, 2002.

Gallin, JI. *Principles and Practice of Clinical Research*, San Diego, CA: Academic Press, 2002.

Jensen, E. *Not Just Another GCP Handbook: A Practical Guide to FDA/DHHS Requirements*, New York, NY: PJB Publications Ltd., 2003. (available at: http://www.pjbpubs.com/cms.asp?pageid=287 &reportid=626)

Loue, S. *Textbook of Research Ethics: Theory and Practice*, New York, N.Y.: Kluwer Academic/Plenum Pub. Corp., 2000.

Penslar, RL, National Institutes of Health (U.S.). Office for Protection from Research Risks. *Protecting Human Research Subjects: Institutional Review Board Guidebook*, 2nd ed. Bethesda, MD; Washington, DC: GPO, 1993.

Shamoo, AE, Khin-Maung-Gyi, FA. *Ethics of the Use of Human Subjects in Research: Practical Guide*, London; New York: Garland Science, 2002.

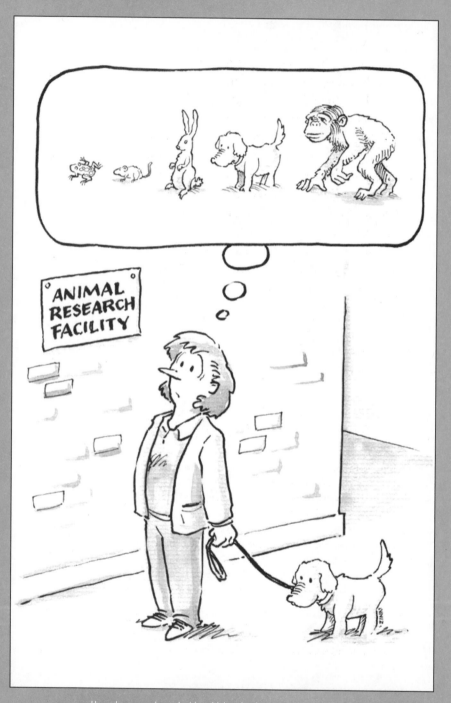

How do researchers decide which animals are used in research?

4. The Welfare of Laboratory Animals

Animal research is as carefully regulated as human research, but for different reasons. With humans, regulation stems from the need to assure that the benefits all humans gain from human research do not impose unacceptable burdens on some research participants. Animals may benefit from the information gained through animal experimentation and some research with animals is conducted specifically for the purpose of improving animal health (veterinary medicine and animal husbandry research). But most animal research is conducted primarily for the benefit of humans, not animals. Moreover, unlike humans, animals cannot consent to participate in experiments or comment on their treatment, creating special needs that should be taken into consideration in their care and use.

The special needs of animals have evolved over time into policies for the appropriate care and use of all animals

Case Study

After many years using fish and frogs to study brain function, Dr. Ruth Q. encountered some problems that can be explored only using new animal models. For the near future, she plans to turn to mice or rats, but eventually may have to do some research using cats or dogs. To help prepare the way for this new research, she decides to put a note about her plans in the progress report for her current research grant, which runs out next year.

The day after she gave a draft of the progress report to her long-time research assistant, he came to her with a troubled look on his face. Although he never told her, the main reason he applied for the job in her laboratory many years ago was the fact that she did not use warm-blooded animals in her research. If she changed her animal models as planned, he would have to quit his job and had no prospects for getting another position that paid as well and was as rewarding.

Does Dr. Q. have any obligation to consider her research assistant's views before she redirects his research?

Why are objections raised to the use of some animals in research and how can those objections be answered?

Why are there more objections to using some animals in research compared to others?

involved in research, research training, and biological testing activities. Researchers can meet their responsibilities by:

✓ knowing what activities are subject to regulation,

✓ understanding and following the rules for project approval,

✓ obtaining appropriate training, and

✓ accepting continuing responsibility for compliance through all stages of a project.

If you expect to use or study living animals in your research, regardless of the level of invasiveness, familiarize yourself with your responsibilities and check with someone in a position of authority before making any plans or undertaking any work.

4a. Rules, policies, and guidelines

The current rules, policies, and professional guidelines for the responsible use of animals in research are the product of roughly 50 years of ongoing discussion between government, the public, animal care professionals, and

---

Animal Welfare Act as Amended (7 USC, 2131-2156)

Section 1.

(a) This Act may be cited as the **"Animal Welfare Act."**

(b) The Congress finds that animals and activities which are regulated under this Act are either in interstate or foreign commerce or substantially affect such commerce or the free flow thereof, and that regulation of animals and activities as provided in this Act is necessary to prevent and eliminate burdens upon such commerce and to effectively regulate such commerce, in order—

(1) to insure that animals intended for use in research facilities or for exhibition purposes or for use as pets are provided humane care and treatment;

(2) to assure the humane treatment of animals during transportation in commerce; and

(3) to protect the owners of animals from the theft of their animals by preventing the sale or use of animals which have been stolen.

http://www.nal.usda.gov/awic/legislat/awa.htm

PHS Policy on Humane Care and Use of Laboratory Animals (Amended, August 2002)

II. Applicability

This Policy is applicable to all PHS-conducted or supported activities involving animals, whether the activities are performed at a PHS agency, an awardee institution, or any other institution and conducted in the United States, the Commonwealth of Puerto Rico, or any territory or possession of the United States.

http://grants2.nih.gov/grants/olaw/references/phspol.htm

researchers. The conclusions reached through these discussions are laid out in two key sources of information for researchers who use animals in their work: Federal regulations and professional guidelines.

Federal regulations. Over the last 50 years, Congress has addressed the responsible use of animals in research on a number of occasions and drafted two important statutes:

✓ the 1966 Animal Welfare Act (revised 1970, 1976, 1985, and 1990) and

✓ the 1985 Health Research Extension Act, Sec. 495.

The former broadly assigns authority for the responsible transportation, care, and use of animals to the United States Department of Agriculture (USDA), as implemented by Title 9 of the Code of Federal Regulations. It covers animals used "in research facilities or for exhibition purposes or for use as pets." The latter law delegates authority for the responsible use of animals in "biomedical and behavioral research" to the Secretary of Health and Human Services (HHS), acting through the Director of the National Institutes of Health (NIH) and the Office of Laboratory Animal Welfare (OLAW), NIH.

Researchers who use animals in research, including observational research, or teaching, can come under the jurisdiction of the USDA animal welfare regulations and/or the PHS Policy on Humane Care and Use of Laboratory Animals (hereafter, PHS Policy), which carries out the provisions of the 1985 Health Research Extension Act. They therefore should be familiar with both.

Guidelines. In the late 1950's, a group of animal-care professionals formed the "Animal Care Panel" (ACP) specifically for the purpose of establishing a professional standard for laboratory animal care and facilities. Their work led to the publication of a comprehensive and influential *Guide for Laboratory Animal Facilities and Care* (1963, revised 1965, 1968, 1972, 1978, 1985, and 1996). The current edition, now called the *Guide for the Care and Use of Laboratory Animals,* or *Guide,* as it is commonly referenced, was prepared by a committee appointed by the National Research Council of the National Academy of Sciences and provides guidance on:

✓ Institutional Policies and Responsibilities;

✓ Animal Environment, Housing, and Management;

Guide for the Care and Use of Laboratory Animals (1996)

The Guide for the Care and Use of Laboratory Animals (the Guide) was first published in 1963 under the title Guide for Laboratory Animal Facilities and Care and was revised in 1965, 1968, 1972, 1978, and 1985. More than 400,000 copies have been distributed since it was first published, and it is widely accepted as a primary reference on animal care and use. The changes and new material in this seventh edition are in keeping with the belief that the Guide is subject to modification with changing conditions and new information.

The purpose of the Guide, as expressed in the charge to the Committee to Revise the Guide for the Care and Use of Laboratory Animals, is to assist institutions in caring for and using animals in ways judged to be scientifically, technically, and humanely appropriate. The Guide is also intended to assist investigators in fulfilling their obligation to plan and conduct animal experiments in accord with the highest scientific, humane, and ethical principles. The recommendations are based on published data, scientific principles, expert opinion, and experience with methods and practices that have proved to be consistent with high-quality, humane animal care and use.

http://www.nap.edu/readingroom/books/labrats/preface.html

✓ Veterinary Medical Care; and

✓ Physical Plant.

The *Guide* is widely accepted by both government and research institutions as the most authoritative source of information on most animal care and use questions. The PHS Policy requires that PHS-funded institutions use the *Guide* as a basis for developing and implementing an institutional program for animal care and use.

4b. Definitions

The term "animal" is defined differently in the statutes, codes, policies, and guidelines that govern animal research. Federally funded research is guided by two key definitions:

✓ The PHS Policy, which applies to all PHS-funded activities involving animals, defines "animals" as "any live, vertebrate animals used or intended for use in research, research training, experimentation, or biological testing or for related purposes."

✓ The Federal Code that implements the Animal Welfare Act (Title 9) covers warm-blooded animals but excludes "[b]irds, rats of the genus Rattus and mice of the genus Mus bred for use in research, and horses not used for research purposes and other farm animals...."

Many institutions apply uniform and consistent standards to all activities involving animals regardless of the source of funding or legal requirements as a way of ensuring broad compliance with all regulations covering the care and use of animals in research.

Researchers are not authorized to make decisions about covered or excluded research themselves. Therefore, anyone who plans to use animals in research, teaching, testing and other covered activities is well advised to assume a broad definition and to consult with their institutional committee (see below) before ordering animals or beginning work.

4c. Institutional organization

The task of assuring that researchers adhere to the regulations and guidelines for the responsible care and use of animals is generally recognized to be an institutional responsibility. Institutions vest authority for animal care and use in an "institutional official" (IO), who in turn appoints the Congressionally mandated Institutional Animal Care and Use Committee (IACUC), administers institutional care and use units at institutions that are large enough to have such, and handles other general matters relating to the care and use of animals at that institution.

IACUCs. Following the provisions of the 1985 Health Research Extension Act, PHS Policy, USDA regulations, the *Guide*, and the Association for Assessment and Accreditation of Laboratory Animal Care (AAALAC) require research institutions to establish an IACUC. IACUCs oversee and evaluate all aspects of the institution's animal program, procedures, and facilities. Its members must include a doctor of veterinary medicine, one researcher who uses animals in research, and one person who is not affiliated with the institution. Many IACUCs also have a researcher who does not use animals or a member who has some grounding in ethics.

IACUC Members are appointed by their institution, but they have considerable independent authority. Their responsibilities include:

✓ reviewing and approving all animal use research proposals,

✓ reviewing the institution's animal care program,

✓ inspecting (at least twice a year) the institution's animal facilities,

✓ receiving and reviewing concerns raised about the care and use of animals, and

✓ submitting reports to the Institutional Official.

IACUCs also have independent authority to suspend projects if they determine that they are not being conducted in accordance with applicable requirements. This authority comes directly from Congress through the Health Research Extension Act and can be exercised independent of any other institutional administrative authority.

Animal care and use units. Research institutions with large animal research programs generally have centralized animal care and use units that provide veterinary support, training in procedures, and advice on analgesics, anesthesia, euthanasia, and occupational health and safety. While the staff employed in these units cannot approve research protocols for the institution or make decisions specifically assigned to the institutional IACUC, as animal care professionals they are an excellent local source of information about the responsible care and use of animals in research.

4d. Federal and voluntary oversight

OLAW, USDA, and a voluntary accreditation program (Association for Assessment and Accreditation of Laboratory Animal Care—AAALAC) are charged with or assume the task of assuring that research institutions live up to their responsibilities for the care and use of animals in research.

OLAW. OLAW relies on an "assurance" mechanism to monitor institutional compliance with the PHS Policy. An "Assurance" is a signed agreement submitted by a research institution confirming that it will:

✓ comply with applicable rules and policies for animal care and use,

✓ provide a description of the institution's program for animal care and use,

✓ maintain an appropriate IACUC, and

✓ appoint a responsible IO for compliance.

The Assurance is considered the cornerstone of a trust relationship between the institution and the PHS and grants considerable authority to institutions for self-regulation.

Association for Assessment and Accreditation of Laboratory Animal Care (AAALAC) International

AAALAC International is a private, nonprofit organization that promotes the humane treatment of animals in science through voluntary accreditation and assessment programs. ...

More than 700 companies, universities, hospitals, government agencies and other research institutions in 29 countries have earned AAALAC accreditation, demonstrating their commitment to responsible animal care and use. These institutions volunteer to participate in AAALAC's program, in addition to complying with the local, state and federal laws that regulate animal research.

http://www.aaalac.org/about/index.cfm

An OLAW-approved Assurance and compliance with PHS policy are considered terms and conditions of receiving PHS funds. Compliance is monitored by OLAW through annual mandatory institutional reporting to OLAW and in the event of noncompliance, serious deviations from the *Guide*, or IACUC suspensions. OLAW conducts limited site visits and reviews, and if necessary conducts investigations of reported noncompliance. Institutions that fail to submit an Assurance or to live up to the terms of their Assurance can have their approval to use animals in research, teaching, and testing suspended.

USDA. The animal welfare regulations also have mandatory reporting requirements, but USDA is an inspection-based system carried out by USDA Veterinary Medical Officers. Rather than allowing institutions to "assure" their own compliance, USDA visits sites, either announced or unannounced, to check whether institutions are in compliance. If violations are found, the institution is then subject to administrative fines and penalties.

Accreditation programs. Animal use programs can be, and most large ones are, accredited by the Association for Assessment and Accreditation of Laboratory Animal Care (AAALAC) International. AAALAC is "a private nonprofit organization that promotes the humane treatment of animals in science through a voluntary accreditation program." It is governed by a Board of Trustees representing scientific, professional, and educational organizations. Its Council on Accreditation is composed of animal care and use professionals and researchers who conduct the program evaluations that determine which institutions are awarded accreditation.

AAALAC relies on widely accepted guidelines, such as the *Guide*, and other peer-reviewed resources when evaluating an institution's animal research program. During the accreditation process, AAALAC accreditors evaluate all aspects of an institution's animal research program. If an institution meets AAALAC's standards, it receives an accreditation for a specified period of time and can use this accreditation to demonstrate its commitment to high standards for the care and use of animals.

4e. Principles for the responsible use of animals in research

There is a range of views about the morality of animal experimentation. Antivivisectionists hold that humans have no right to place their own welfare above the welfare of animals and therefore all animal experimentation is immoral. Many animal welfare organizations find that some scientifically necessary experimentation is acceptable, but that it should be kept to a minimum and conducted on animals low on the phylogenetic scale, in ways that minimize pain and suffering. Many scientists feel that extensive animal experimentation is necessary and moral, provided it is based on sound scientific practices and utilizes quality animal care, along with minimization of pain and distress.

To help researchers and IACUCs make decisions about the responsible and appropriate use of animals in research, the Federal government has adopted nine *Principles for the Utilization and Care of Vertebrate Animals used in Testing, Research, and Training* (see box, next page). These principles specify requirements for planning and conducting research and are useful to investigators and IACUCs. When questions arise, PHS policy and USDA regulations provide further criteria for researchers and IACUCs to consider in assessing protocols.

Further practical advice on ways to assure appropriate respect for animals can be found in the "three Rs of alternatives" devised by Russell and Burch in 1959:

✓ Replacement—using non-animal models such as microorganisms or cell culture techniques, computer simulations, or species lower on the phylogenetic scale.

✓ Reduction—using methods aimed at reducing the numbers of animals such as minimization of variability, appropriate selection of animal model, minimization of animal loss, and careful experimental design.

✓ Refinement—the elimination or reduction of unnecessary pain and distress.

US Government Principles for the Utilization and Care of Vertebrate Animals Used in Testing, Research, and Training

[Researchers should:]

1. follow the rules and regulations for the transportation, care, and use of animals;

2. design and perform research with consideration of relevance to human or animal health, the advancement of knowledge, or the good of society;

3. use appropriate species, quality, and the minimum number of animals to obtain valid results, and consider non-animal models;

4. avoid or minimize pain, discomfort, and distress when consistent with sound scientific practices;

5. use appropriate sedation, analgesia, or anesthesia;

6. painlessly kill animals that will suffer severe or chronic pain or distress that cannot be relieved;

7. feed and house animals appropriately and provide veterinary care as indicated;

8. assure that everyone who is responsible for the care and treatment of animals during the research is appropriately qualified and trained; and

9. defer any exceptions to these principles to the appropriate IACUC.

http://grants.nih.gov/grants/olaw/references/phspol.htm#USGovPrinciples/

Although PHS Policy is not explicit in addressing refinements, the requirements to use appropriate animal models and numbers of animals and to avoid or minimize pain and distress are, for all practical purposes, synonymous with requirements to consider alternative methods that reduce, refine, or replace the use of animals. USDA animal welfare regulations require a written narrative of the methods used and sources consulted to determine the availability of alternatives.

Knowing the concerns society has about the use of animals in research, researchers should be prepared to explain why they are using a particular species in their research; why pain or discomfort cannot be avoided; why it may be necessary to sacrifice the animals; and why non-animal options cannot be used to gather the same information or to achieve the same ends, based on the principles set out in the *U.S. Government Principles* and other sources of guidance.

4f. Broader responsibilities

Even with all of the care and review that currently is used to assure the responsible use of animals in research, animal research is still controversial and raises concerns that cannot easily be set aside.

Pain and suffering. Some experimental information cannot be gained without subjecting animals to pain and suffering. Researchers who study the effects of severe trauma, such as child abuse, can learn a great deal about physiological change by subjecting animals to different levels of pain and suffering. This can be done by administering mild electric shocks, forcing animals such as rats to swim until they reach exhaustion, or subjecting them to other traumatic treatments. How much pain and suffering is acceptable in experiments is not easily determined.

Concern for different species. There is widespread agreement that some animals, such as primates and household pets, deserve more protection than other animals, such as worms and clams. There is less agreement about the relative protection that is needed for species within general groups of animals, such as cats, dogs, pigs, rabbits, mice, and rats. What moral considerations set one species apart from another when making decisions about the use to which it can be put in experiments?

Unnecessary experiments. Members of the public disagree about the use to which animals can reasonably be put in research, testing, and teaching. Animals are used to test the safety of experimental drugs, but should they also be used to test the toxicity of chemicals or cosmetics (as once was common, but has largely been abandoned)? Should they be used to train surgeons to do elective surgery? Do researchers sometimes use more animals in an experiment than is absolutely necessary or use animals when other means of testing would provide the same information?

Discussions about the responsible use of animals in research are not likely to dissipate in the near future. If animals are essential to your research and cannot be replaced; if you cannot reduce the number without compromising the experiment; and if you cannot further refine your methods to reduce pain and suffering, then presumably you have done all you can to meet your responsibility. However, do not forget that society does not have to permit the use of animals in research. It can seek to protect animals through complex and expensive regulations if it loses confidence in the research community's ability to regulate itself.

Questions for discussion

1. Should all animals used in research be treated the same or are there reasons to treat some animals differently than others?

2. Are there some animals that should not be used in research?

3. What circumstances justify pain and suffering of experimental animals?

4. How should research animals be procured? How should they be housed and treated during experiments?

5. How should members of IACUCs be selected? What constituencies should be represented on IACUCs?

Resources

Policies, Reports, and Policy Statements

National Academy of Sciences. Institute of Laboratory Animal Resources Commission of Life Sciences. *Guide for the Care and Use of Laboratory Animals*, Washington, DC: National Academy Press, 1996. (available at: http://www.nap.edu/readingroom/books/labrats/)

National Institutes of Health. *U.S. Government Principles for the Utilization and Care of Vertebrate Animals Used in Testing, Research, and Training*, Bethesda, MD: National Institutes of Health, nd. (available at: http://grants.nih.gov/grants/olaw/references/phspol.htm#USGovPrinciples)

Public Health Service. *Public Health Service Policy on Humane Care and Use of Laboratory Animals*, Washington, DC: GPO, 2002. (available at: http://grants2.nih.gov/grants/olaw/references/phspol.htm)

United States. Congress. *Animal Welfare Act*, PL 89-544, 1966. (available at: http://www.nal.usda.gov/awic/legislat/awa.htm)

United States Department of Agriculture. *USDA Animal and Plant Health Inspection Animal Care Policy Manual*, Washington, DC: GPO, nd. (available at: http://www.aphis.usda.gov/ac/polmanpdf.html)

General Information Web Sites

Association for the Assessment and Accreditation of Laboratory Animal Care. *Home Page*. http://www.aaalac.org/

National Institutes of Health. Office of Laboratory Animals Welfare. *Home Page*. http://grants2.nih.gov/grants/olaw/olaw.htm

United States Department of Agriculture. Animal Care Program. *Home Page*. http://www.aphis.usda.gov/ac/

Additional Reading

Baird, RM, Rosenbaum, SE. *Animal Experimentation: The Moral Issues*, Buffalo, NY: Prometheus Books, 1991.

Gluck, JP, DiPasquale, T, Orlans, FB. *Applied Ethics in Animal Research: Philosophy, Regulation, and Laboratory Applications*, West Lafayette, IN: Purdue University Press, 2002.

Hart, LA. *Responsible Conduct with Animals in Research*, New York: Oxford University Press, 1998.

Monamy, V. *Animal Experimentation: A Guide to the Issues*, Cambridge, United Kingdom; New York: Cambridge University Press, 2000.

Paul, EF, Paul, J. *Why Animal Experimentation Matters: The Use of Animals in Medical Research*, New Studies in Social Policy, New Brunswick, NJ: Social Philosophy and Policy Foundation: Transaction, 2001.

Rudacille, D. *The Scalpel and the Butterfly: The War Between Animal Research and Animal Protection*, New York: Farrar, Straus and Giroux, 2000.

Russell, WMS, Burch, RL. *The Principles of Humane Animal Experimental Technique*, London: Methuen, 1959.

Smith, CP, Animal Welfare Information Center (U.S.). *Animal Welfare and Ethics: Resources for Youth and College Agricultural Educators*, Revised and enlarged ed. *AWIC resource series; no. 6*, Beltsville, MD: U.S. Department of Agriculture Agricultural Research Service National Agricultural Library Animal Welfare Information Center, 2000.

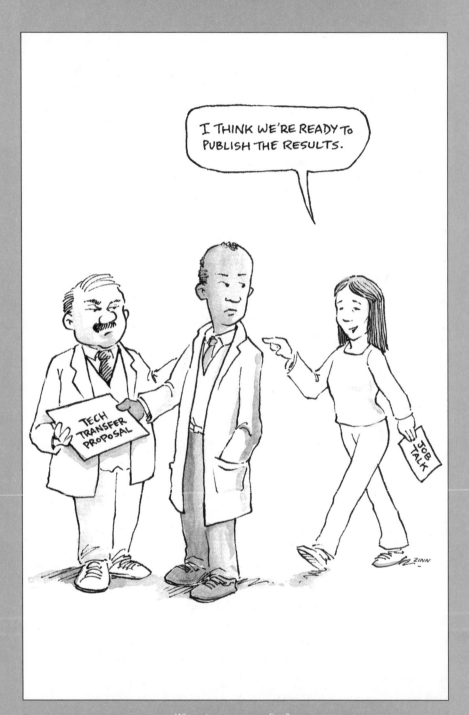

Whose interest comes first?

5. Conflicts of Interest

Researchers work hard, often spending long hours and sometimes weekends in the laboratory, library, or at professional meetings. Their motivation for working hard stems from many sources. Research:

✓ advances knowledge,

✓ leads to discoveries that will benefit individuals and society,

✓ furthers professional advancement, and/or

✓ results in personal gain and satisfaction.

Each of these incentives or *interests* is commonly recognized as responsible and justifiable.

Researchers are allowed to and even encouraged to profit from their work (see the discussion of the Bayh-Dole Act, below). Professional advancement as a researcher depends on productivity. Society expects researchers to use the

Case Study

Early in his undergraduate education, Dr. Sam M. decided to dedicate his studies to finding a cure for a psychological disorder that seemed to run in his family. As a biology major, he pursued independent research projects and worked long hours as a lab assistant. He then enrolled in a PhD program in psychopharmacology and is now completing a 3-year postdoc in the neurosciences.

During his postdoc he worked on a promising compound he first discovered during his graduate years. His work has gone well and he feels the time is right to explore clinical applications. After more than a decade of living on student and postdoc wages, he is also ready for a better paying job.

As Sam weighs the options of an academic versus an industry job, he begins to wonder about who owns or will own the useful applications of his work, if and when there are any. Will it be owned by:

his graduate institution, where he first worked on the promising compound?

his postdoc institution, where he refined his ideas?

his future academic or industry employer?

himself, based on his hard work and innovative ideas?

society, which funded parts of his education and most of his research?

Who has a legitimate interest in Sam's work and when do his own personal financial interests create a conflict of interest?

funds it supplies to advance knowledge and to make useful discoveries. Personal gain and satisfaction provide strong incentives for doing a good job and acting responsibly.

Researchers' interests can and often do conflict with one another. The advancement of knowledge is usually best served by sharing ideas with colleagues, putting many minds to work on the same problem. But personal gain is sometimes best served by keeping ideas to oneself until they are fully developed and then protected through patents, copyrights, or publications. Legitimate research interests can create competing responsibilities and lead to what is commonly called *conflicts of interest.*

It is important to understand that *conflicts of interest* are not inherently wrong. The complex and demanding nature of research today inevitably gives rise to competing obligations and interests. Researchers are expected to serve on committees, to train young researchers, to teach, and to review grants and manuscripts at the same time they pursue their own research. Conflicts of interest cannot and need not be avoided. However, in three crucial areas:

✓ financial gain,

✓ work commitments, and

✓ intellectual and personal matters,

special steps are needed to assure that conflicts do not interfere with the responsible practice of research.

5a. Financial conflicts

Personal interests and the prospect of financial gain should not, but unfortunately can, improperly influence a researcher's fundamental obligation to truth and honesty. Although researchers should not, they can find ways to delay unfairly a competitor's work in order to secure a patent or some other financial advantage for themselves. Financial interests can provide a strong incentive to overemphasize or underemphasize research findings or even to engage in research misconduct (Chapter 2). *Financial conflicts of interest* are situations that create perceived or actual tensions between personal financial gain and adherence to the fundamental values of honesty, accuracy, efficiency, and objectivity (Section I).

Financial interests are not inherently wrong. Researchers are permitted to benefit financially from their work. A 1980 Congressional law known as the Bayh-Dole Act encourages researchers and research institutions to use copyrights, patents, and licenses to put research ideas to use for the good of the public. Prior to this time, there were no uniform policies regulating the ownership of ideas developed with public funding. Bayh-Dole essentially gives that ownership to research institutions as an incentive to put ideas to work for the overall good of society. It not only approves of but, in fact, strongly encourages researchers and research institutions to have financial interests as a way of ensuring that the public's investment in research is used to stimulate economic growth.

While financial interests should not and in most instances do not compromise intellectual honesty, they certainly can, especially if the financial interests are *significant.*

Bayh-Dole Act (Public Law: 96-517)
Policy and Objective
35 USC Part II, Chapter 18, Section 200

It is the policy and objective of the Congress to use the patent system to promote the utilization of inventions arising from federally supported research and development efforts; to promote collaboration between commercial concerns and nonprofit organizations, including universities; to ensure that inventions made by nonprofit organizations and small business firms are used in a manner to promote free competition and enterprise without unduly encumbering future research and discovery; to promote the commercialization and public availability of inventions made in the United States by United States industry and labor; to ensure that the Government obtains sufficient rights in federally supported inventions to meet the needs of the Government and protect the public against nonuse or unreasonable use of inventions; and to minimize the costs of administering policies in this area.

http://www.law.cornell.edu/uscode/html/uscode35/usc_sup_01_35_10_II_20_18.html

Universities are currently starting hundreds of new businesses based on researchers' ideas. Some of these businesses will generate significant profits (hundreds of thousands to millions of dollars each year). If the difference between commercial success and failure rests on one key publication, the pressure to put the best face on that publication can be considerable.

Financial conflicts also arise from the ever-present pressure researchers have to secure funds to support their research. A private sponsor might withdraw support from a project if it does not produce the "right" results. Success in the stiff competition for research grants can rest on having the "right" preliminary results. Research is expensive, funding often in short supply. The pressure simply to survive, much less profit personally, can and does create financial conflicts of interest.

Federal policies. Concerns about the actual or potential adverse effect of financial interests on research prompted the Public Health Service (PHS) and the National Science Foundation (NSF) to adopt conflict of interest policies in the mid-1990's. These policies require research institutions to establish administrative procedures for:

✓ reporting *significant* conflicts before any research is undertaken;

✓ managing, reducing, or eliminating *significant* financial conflicts of interest; and

✓ providing subsequent information on how the conflicts were handled.

Significant financial conflict is defined as:

✓ additional earnings in excess of $10,000 a year, or

✓ equity interests in excess of 5 percent in an entity that stands to benefit from the research.

The financial interests of all immediate family members are included in these figures.

Department of Health and Human Services
Conflict of Interest Definitions
45 CFR 94.3

Significant Financial Interest means anything of monetary value, including but not limited to, salary or other payments for services (e.g., consulting fees or honoraria); equity interests (e.g., stocks, stock options or other ownership interests); and intellectual property rights (e.g., patents, copyrights and royalties from such rights). The term does not include:

(1) Salary, royalties, or other remuneration from the applicant institution;

(2) Any ownership interests in the institution, if the institution is an applicant under the SBIR program;

(3) Income from seminars, lectures, or teaching engagements sponsored by public or nonprofit entities;

(4) Income from service on advisory committees or review panels for public or nonprofit entities;

(5) An equity interest that when aggregated for the Investigator and the Investigator's spouse and dependent children, meets both of the following tests: Does not exceed $10,000 in value as determined through reference to public prices or other reasonable measures of fair market value, and does not represent more than a five percent owner-ship interest in any single entity; or

(6) Salary, royalties or other payments that when aggregated for the investigator and the investigator's spouse and dependent children over the next twelve months, are not reasonably expected to exceed $10,000.

http://a257.g.akamaitech.net/7/257/2422/14mar20010800/edocket.access.gpo.gov/cfr_2002/octqtr/45cfr94.3.htm

State and local policies. Although the Federal requirements apply only to PHS- and NSF-funded research, many research institutions have adopted global policies that apply to all researchers. Many also use different values for defining *significant,* to as low as any financial interest. Researchers therefore should check their local conflict-of-interest policy to find out when and what they are required to report. They also need to keep in mind that many states have their own conflict-of-interest policies, which apply to all state-paid employees.

AAMC Task Force Recommendations
Financial Conflicts of Interest in Clinical Research
(December 2001)

B. In the event of compelling circumstances, an individual holding significant financial interests in human subjects research may be permitted to conduct the research. Whether the circumstances are deemed compelling will depend in each case upon the nature of the science, the nature of the interest, how closely the interest is related to the research, and the degree to which the interest may be affected by, the research....

C. Institutional policies should require full prior reporting of each covered individual's significant financial interests that would reasonably appear to be affected by the individual's research, updated reporting of any relevant change in financial circumstances, and review of any significant financial interests in a research project by the institution's COI committee prior to final IRB approval of the research. COI committee findings and determinations should inform the IRB's review of any research protocol or proposal, although the IRB may require additional safeguards or demand reduction or elimination of the financial interest....

http://www.aamc.org/research/coi/firstreport.pdf

New England Journal of Medicine
Conflict of Interest Policy
June 13, 2002

[B]eginning with this issue of the Journal, we have modified the statement in Information for Authors to read as follows:

> Because the essence of reviews and editorials is selection and interpretation of the literature, the Journal expects that authors of such articles will not have any significant financial interest in a company (or its competitor) that makes a product discussed in the article.

The addition of the word "significant" acknowledges that not all financial associations are the same. Some, such as the receipt of honorariums for occasional educational lectures sponsored by biomedical companies, may be appropriately viewed as minor and unlikely to influence an author's judgment. Others, such as ownership of substantial equity in a company, are of greater concern. It is our intent to focus on the financial relationships that, in our judgment, could produce bias, or the perception of bias, in an article.

http://content.nejm.org/cgi/content/full/346/24/1901

Professional societies and journal policies.
A number of professional societies have issued reports
or made recommendations on appropriate ways to handle
conflicts of interest. Similarly, more and more journals now
require researchers to disclose real or potential financial
conflicts. Sometimes disclosure must be made to the journal
editor, who decides what, if any, action is needed. Sometimes
disclosures must be included in the publication itself. Before
submitting an article to a journal for publication, researchers
should carefully check and make sure they have followed
that publication's conflict of interest policies.

5b. Conflicts of commitment

Conflicts of commitment arise from situations that place
competing demands on researchers' time and loyalties. At
any time, a researcher might be:

✓ working on one or more funded projects;

✓ preparing to submit a request for a new project;

✓ teaching and advising students;

✓ attending professional meetings and giving lectures;

✓ serving as a peer reviewer;

✓ sitting on advisory boards; or

✓ working as a paid consultant, officer, or employee in a private
company.

Each of these activities requires time and makes demands
on a researcher's institutional commitments. Care needs
to be taken to assure that these commitments do not
inappropriately interfere with one another.

Allocation of time. Researchers must be careful to
follow rules for the allocation of time. Federally funded
researchers must follow the rules for cost accounting
published by the Office of Management and Budget
in a document known as *Circular A-21*. Most research

institutions also have rules for how researchers spend their time, particularly time serving as paid consultants, giving paid lectures, or working as an employee in a private company. At a minimum, these rules require that researchers:

✓ honor time commitments they have made, such as devoting a specified percentage of time to a grant or contract;

✓ refrain from charging two sources of funding for the same time; and

✓ seek advice if they are unsure whether a particular commitment of time is allowed under an institution's or the Federal Government's policies.

Although researchers will frequently work on several projects at the same time, in the final analysis primary work obligations must be met. In addition, the time devoted to one project ordinarily cannot be billed to another.

Relationships with students. Academic researchers involved in start-up ventures often have opportunities to hire students. This puts them in a situation where they can hire their own students. As mentors, they have a primary obligation to help students develop into independent researchers. As heads of start-up companies, their primary obligation is to see promising ideas commercialized. While the two responsibilities can complement one another, they can also be in conflict. Should an individual who is both the researcher's student and employee be advised to develop a promising idea that could lead to an independent career or to work on a more routine problem that will benefit the start-up company? Situations such as these create conflicts and should be avoided or appropriately managed.

Use of resources. Equipment and supplies purchased with public funds can easily be used to advance private research interests. While this might seem like a harmless practice, particularly if the equipment is not in constant use, unless a researcher has permission to use the equipment to support private research, this practice is not

Stanford University
Conflict of Commitment Policy

1. Outside consulting privileges are not normally available to Academic Staff. They may consult only with permission, as noted below. Under no circumstances may any Academic Staff member's outside consulting work exceed the limits imposed by the faculty consulting policy, i.e., 13 days per calendar quarter (that is, one day in seven) on a full-time equivalent basis.... Academic Staff may not use University resources, including facilities, personnel, equipment, or confidential information, except in a purely incidental way, as part of any outside consulting activities nor for any other purposes that are unrelated to the mission of the University.

2. Academic Staff must maintain a significant presence on campus (main or overseas) throughout each quarter in which they are employed by Stanford, consistent with the scope of their appointment.

3. Academic Staff must not allow other professional activities to detract from their primary allegiance to Stanford. For example, Academic Staff employed on a full-time basis must not have significant outside managerial responsibilities nor act as a principal investigator on sponsored projects that could be conducted at Stanford University but instead are submitted and managed through another institution.

http://www.stanford.edu/dept/DoR/rph/4-4.html

appropriate. The equipment can be used for other university work since this is allowed by the government. But it cannot be used for a personal project without permission. It also cannot be used for research that is explicitly prohibited by the Federal government, such as stem cell research using lines not authorized by the President's policy.

Disclosure of affiliations. It is widely agreed that outside affiliations that create conflicts of interest should be listed on academic publications, but should researchers list their academic affiliations on other publications? As president or CEO of a new company, is it appropriate for a researcher to also note in the end-of-the-year financial report that she or he is also a full professor at a prestigious university? Should researchers who serve on private boards list their academic affiliation? Researchers must be careful to separate their academic or institutional work from their private work. In particular, they should not inappropriately use their institutional research affiliation to advance their private interests by implying, for example, that private work has the support of their research institution if it does not.

Representing outside entities. The results researchers commercialize in private ventures, such as drugs used in a university hospital, a software program used in an accounting office, or a consultation service for employees, might be used by their primary employer. In these cases, the researcher could be the resident expert on the goods and services in question. Each employer in this case presumably wants the best deal on the goods and services, whereas the researcher is also interested in personal profits, creating a conflict of commitment.

Since the situations described above are often not subject to specific policies or guidance, judgments about responsible conduct often rest with the researcher. In making judgments about the best way to deal with institutional conflicts, it is helpful to take into consideration:

✓ how others will view your commitments and

✓ the judgment of someone who has no stake in the outcome.

In addition, it is always a good idea, even if it is not required, to seek advice from an institutional official.

5c. Personal and intellectual conflicts

Researchers are also expected to avoid bias in proposing, conducting, reporting, and reviewing research. They therefore should be careful to avoid making judgments or presenting conclusions based solely on personal opinion or affiliations rather than on scientific evidence.

Personal conflicts are usually the easiest to identify and resolve. Researchers generally should not serve as reviewers for grants and publications submitted by close colleagues and students. Their presumed *interest* in seeing their colleagues and students succeed could conflict with their obligation to makes judgments based solely on the evidence at hand. Most granting agencies require reviewers to disclose conflicts of interest, including personal conflicts, as a condition of service.

Intellectual conflicts are more difficult to identify, but are nonetheless important. If a researcher holds strong personal views on the importance of a particular area of research or set of research findings, those views should be disclosed so that others can take them into consideration when judging the researcher's statements. The same is true of strong moral convictions that could influence a researcher's scientific opinions. This is particularly true when researchers serve as expert witnesses or advisors. It is for precisely this reason that the National Academy of Sciences, which has provided essential science advice to the Federal Government since the Civil War, carefully considers all conflicts of interest when it sets up advisory panels (see box, below).

Federal Advisory Committee Act
Public Disclosure Requirements Applicable to the
National Academy of Sciences
January 5, 1997

The Academy shall determine and provide public notice of the names and brief biographies of individuals that the Academy appoints or intends to appoint to serve on the committee. The Academy shall determine and provide a reasonable opportunity for the public to comment on such appointments before they are made or, if the Academy determines such prior comment is not practicable, in the period immediately following the appointments. The Academy shall make its best efforts to ensure that (A) no individual appointed to serve on the committee has a conflict of interest that is relevant to the functions to be performed, unless such conflict is promptly and publicly disclosed and the Academy determines that the conflict is unavoidable, (B) the committee membership is fairly balanced as determined by the Academy to be appropriate for the functions to be performed, and (C) the final report of the Academy will be the result of the Academy's independent judgment. The Academy shall require that individuals that the Academy appoints or intends to appoint to serve on the committee inform the Academy of the individual's conflicts of interest that are relevant to the functions to be performed.

http://www.nasonline.org/site/PageServer?pagename = ABOUT_FACA

5d. Reporting and managing significant conflicts

If a researcher has a significant conflict of interest, as defined by Federal, state, institutional, journal, or other policies, it must be reported and managed or eliminated. "Managing" a conflict means finding a way to assure that the interests do not adversely influence the research. Some options for managing conflicts of interest include:

✓ requiring full disclosure of all interests so that others are aware of potential conflicts and can act accordingly;

✓ monitoring the research or checking research results for accuracy and objectivity; or

✓ removing the person with the conflict from crucial steps in the research process, such as the interpretation of data or participating in a particular review decision.

These and other options are either worked out by a conflict of interest review committee or an administrator charged with overseeing conflicts of interest.

If the conflicts cannot be managed and could have an adverse impact on the research, then they must be eliminated, by divesting equity, reducing the income received from the research, assigning supervisory responsibilities to someone else, stepping out of the room when a particular proposal is discussed, or some other action.

Finally, it is important to note that research administrators, funding agencies, journal editors, and conflict of interest committees, not the researcher, should make final decisions about the management of conflicts of interest. This protects the researcher from charges of acting in her or his own interest and helps assure that the most responsible decisions are made.

Questions for discussion

1. Is $10,000 or a 5 percent equity stake an appropriate level for raising concerns about possible conflicts of interest or should other values be used?

2. Should researchers be allowed/encouraged to profit personally from their research apart from their normal compensation?

3. What are appropriate mechanisms for managing financial conflicts of interest?

4. What are appropriate mechanisms for protecting students from a mentor's conflict of commitment?

5. What are appropriate mechanisms for managing intellectual and personal conflicts of interest?

Resources

Policies, Reports, and Policy Statements

Association of American Medical Colleges. *Guidelines for Dealing with Faculty Conflicts of Commitment and Conflicts of Interest in Research*, Washington, DC: AAMC, 1990. (available at: http://www.iit.edu/departments/csep/codes/coe/assoc.amer.medical. colleges.guidelines.html)

_____. *Protecting Subjects, Preserving Trust, Promoting Progress II: Principles and Recommendations for Oversight of an Institution's Financial Interests in Human Subjects Research*, Washington, DC: AAMC, 2002. (available at: http://www.aamc.org/research/coi/ start.htm)

Association of American Medical Colleges, Task Force on Financial Conflicts of Interest in Clinical Research. *Protecting Subjects, Preserving Trust, Promoting Progress–Policy and Guidelines for Oversight of Individual Financial Interests in Human Subjects Research*, Washington, DC: AAMC, 2001. (available at: http:// www.aamc.org/research/coi/start.htm)

Association of American Universities. *Report on Individual and Institutional Financial Conflict of Interest*, Washington, DC: AAU, 2001. (available at: http://www.aau.edu/research/COI.01.pdf)

Council on Government Relations. *Recognizing and Managing Personal Conflicts of Interest*, Washington, DC: COGR, 2002. (available at: http://www.cogr.edu/docs/COIFinal.pdf)

Department of Health and Human Services. *Final Guidance Document: Financial Relationships and Interests in Research Involving Human Subjects: Guidance for Human Subject Protection*, Washington, DC: HHS, 2001. (available at: http://www. hhs.gov/ohrp/humansubjects/finreltn/fguid.pdf)

Drazen, JM, Curfman, GD. "Financial Associations of Authors," *The New England Journal of Medicine* 346, 24 (2002): 1901-1902. (available at: http://content.nejm.org/cgi/content/full/346/24/1901/)

Food and Drug Administration. *Guidance: Financial Disclosure by Clinical Investigators*, Washington, DC: FDA, 2001. (available at: http://www.fda.gov/oc/guidance/financialdis.html)

Institute of Medicine. National Academies of Science. *Study Conduct: Bias and Conflict of Interest*, Washington, DC: IOM, nd. (available at: http://www.iom.edu/subpage.asp?id=5350%0D)

National Institutes of Health. "Objectivity in Research," *Federal Register* 60, 132 (1995): 35809-35819. (available at: http://grants2.nih.gov/grants/guide/notice-files/not95-179.html)

National Science Foundation. "Investigator Financial Disclosure Policy," *Federal Register* 60, 132 (1995): 35820. (available at: http://www.nsf.gov/pubs/stis1996/iin118/iin118.txt)

Office of Management and Budget. *Circular A-21*, Washington, DC: OMB, 2000. (available at: http://www.whitehouse.gov/omb/ circulars/a021/a021.html)

United States, Congress. 105th Congress. First Session. *Federal Advisory Committee Act Amendments of 1997*, PL 105-153 (1997). (available at: http://www.nasonline.org/site/PageServer?pagenam e=ABOUT_FACA)

General Information Web Sites

Association of American Universities. *Conflict of Interest and Misconduct*. http://www.aau.edu/research/conflict.cfm

Association of University Technology Managers. *Home Page*. http://www.autm.net/index_ie.html

National Institutes of Health. Office of Extramural Research. *Conflict of Interest*. http://grants1.nih.gov/grants/policy/coi/

Additional Reading

Boyd, EA, Bero, LA. "Assessing Faculty Financial Relationships With Industry: A Case Study," *Journal of the American Medical Association* 284 (2000): 2209-2214.

Campbell, TID. "Understanding the Potential for Misconduct in University-industry Relationships: An Empirical Study." In *Perspectives on Scholarly Misconduct in the Sciences*, edited by John M. Braxton, 259-282. Columbus, OH: Ohio State University Press, 1999.

Cho, MK, Shohara, R, Schissel, A, Rennie, D. "Policies on Faculty Conflicts of Interest at US Universities," *Journal of the American Medical Association* 284 (2000): 2203-2208.

Jefferson, T, Smith, R, Yee, Y, Drummond, M, Pratt, M, Gale, R. "Evaluating the BMJ Guidelines for Economic Submissions: Prospective Audit of Economic Submissions to BMJ and The Lancet," *Journal of the American Medical Association* 280, 3 (1998): 275-277.

National Institutes of Health. *Financial Conflict of Interest and Research Objectivity: Issues for Investigators and Institutional Review Boards*, Washington, DC: NIH, 2000. (available at: http:// grants1.nih.gov/grants/guide/notice-files/NOT-OD-00-040.html)

Shamoo, AE. "Role of Conflict of Interest in Scientific Objectivity: A Case of a Nobel Prize Work," *Accountability in Research* 2, 1 (1992): 55-75.

United States. Congress. House. Committee on Government Operations. Human Resources and Intergovernmental Relations Subcommittee. *Federal Response to Misconduct in Science, Are Conflicts of Interest Hazardous to our Health?: Hearing before a Subcommittee of the Committee on Government Operations, House of Representatives, One Hundredth Congress, second session, September 29, 1988*, Washington: U.S. G.P.O., 1989.

Part III.

Conducting Research

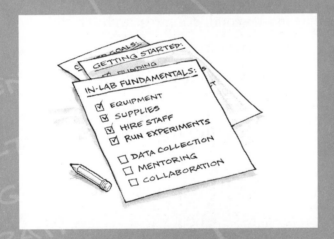

Part III: Conducting Research

ONCE PLANNING IS COMPLETE, RESEARCHERS CAN

finally get on with the work they presumably

enjoy most—conducting research. This is when

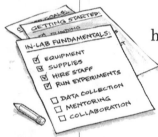

hypotheses and new techniques are

finally tested, when efforts get

underway to solve problems and

put new information to use. At this stage in

any research project, three additional areas

of responsibility become important:

Chapter 6, Data Management Practices, discusses how researchers should collect, store, protect, and share data, mindful of the need to maintain its integrity, validity, and accuracy. Ownership issues must be considered. Some data must be shared with colleagues; other data must be protected from unapproved use. Some data must be preserved for specified periods of time; some destroyed to protect confidentiality.

Chapter 7, Mentor and Trainee Responsibilities, covers the role of the researcher as teacher. The continued growth of research in all fields is vitally dependent upon a constant supply of well-trained researchers. New researchers learn many of the techniques of their profession as they work side by side with established researchers. Established researchers therefore should take their responsibilities as mentors seriously.

Chapter 8, Collaborative Research, explores special responsibilities that arise when researchers work with colleagues, whether in their own discipline or in other disciplines, at other institutions, and in other countries. When collaborating with colleagues, how should intellectual property agreements be worked out? Which country or institution's research policies should be followed? How should project funds and project responsibilities be managed?

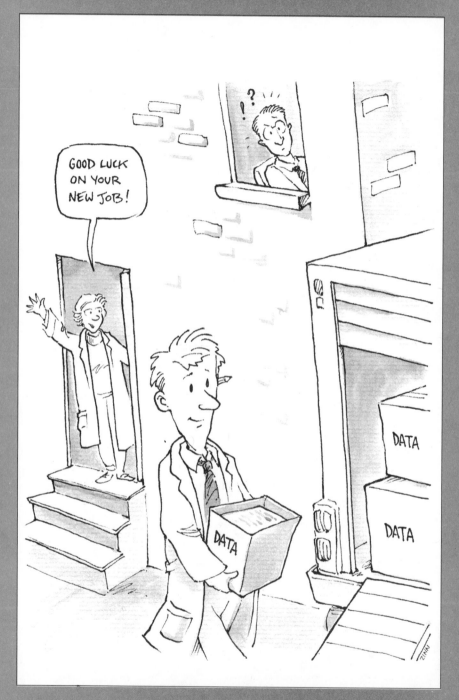

Who owns research data?

6. Data Management Practices

Researchers spend much of their time collecting data. Data are used to confirm or reject hypotheses, to identify new areas of investigation, to guide the development of new investigative techniques, and more. We launch space probes to collect data that help us understand the origins of the universe and use gene databases as tools for understanding and curing disease. Science as we know and practice it today cannot exist without data.

Data management practices are becoming increasingly complex and should be addressed before any data are collected by taking into consideration four important issues:

✓ ownership,

✓ collection,

✓ storage, and

✓ sharing.

The integrity of data and, by implication, the usefulness of the research it supports, depends on careful attention to detail, from initial planning through final publication.

Case Study

Dr. Marion W. long ago learned that good data management practices are essential to responsible research. She therefore carefully supervises the work of her assistants and students, checking notebooks, backing up computer files, and from time to time verifing results for herself.

As she is wrapping up work on one project before starting another, the technology transfer officer at her university calls. A graduate student who previously worked in her laboratory has moved to another university and filed a patent for work that may have been done in Dr. W.'s laboratory on her research funds? If this is the case, the graduate student may not be able to lay claim to the patent.

What records will Dr. W. need to prove that the work was done in her laboratory?

Who owns and controls the data collected in her laboratory?

Do computer records pose any unique problems in this case?

6a. Data ownership

Research produces data. As a product, common sense might suggest that the person who conducts the research should own the product—the data. In fact, conditions imposed by funders, research institutions, and data sources may dictate otherwise.

Funders. Funders provide support for research for different reasons. Government is interested in improving the general health and welfare of society. Private companies are interested in profits, along with benefits to society. Philanthropic organizations are interested in advancing particular causes. These different interests translate into different ownership claims. Typically:

✓ Government gives research institutions the right to use data collected with public funds as an incentive to put research to use for the public good (see the discussion of the Bayh-Dole Act, Chapter 5).

✓ Private companies seek to retain the right to the commercial use of data.

✓ Philanthropic organizations retain or give away ownership rights depending on their interests.

Since the claims of funders can and do vary considerably, researchers must be aware of their obligations to them before they begin collecting data.

With government funding, it is important to distinguish between grants and contracts. Under grants, research-ers must carry out the research as planned and submit reports, but control of the data remains with the institution that received the funds (see below). Contracts require the researcher to deliver a product or service, which is then usually owned and controlled by the government. If your research is supported with government funds, make sure you know whether you are working under a grant or a contract. The difference is significant and could determine who has the right to publish and use your results.

University of Pittsburgh
Guidelines on Data Retention and Access

Data Ownership and Access to Data

Both the principal investigator and the University have responsibilities, and hence, rights concerning access to, use of, and maintenance of original research data. Research data belongs to the University of Pittsburgh, which can be held accountable for the integrity of the data even after the researchers have left the University. Although the primary data should remain in the laboratory where it originated (and hence at the University), consistent with the precepts of academic freedom and intellectual integrity, the investigator may be allowed to retain the research records and materials created by him/her. In the event that the investigator leaves the University, an Agreement on Disposition of Research Data may be negotiated by the investigator and the Department Chair or Dean to allow transfer of research records. However, consistent with the same precepts, it should be specified in the agreement that the University has the right of access to all research records and materials for a reasonable cause after reasonable prior notice regardless of the location of the responsible investigator....

Some circumstances may warrant an exception, requiring that the primary data be retained by the University....

Split of collaborative team: When a collaborative team is dissolved, University of Pittsburgh policy states that each member of the team should have continuing access to the data and materials with which he/she had been working, unless some other agreement was established at the outset. The unique materials prepared in the course of the research should be available/accessible under negotiated terms of a transfer agreement.

http://www.pitt.edu/ ~ provost/retention.html

Research institutions. Support for research is typically awarded to research institutions, not to individual researchers. As the recipients of research funds, research institutions have responsibilities for budgets, regulatory compliance, contractual obligations, and data management. To assure that they are able to meet these responsibilities, research institutions claim ownership rights over data collected with funds given to the institution. This means that researchers cannot automatically assume that they can take their data with them if they move to another institution. The research institution that received the funds may have rights and obligations to retain control over the data.

Data sources. Increasingly research subjects and other entities that are the source of data are seeking some control over data derived from them. Countries with unique resources, such as tropical rain forests, individuals with rare medical conditions, and entities with unique databases, have at one time or another claimed ownership of research results based on their data. Research subjects and entities that have or can be the source of important data may no longer be willing to provide or be the source of data without some ownership stake in the end results.

Well before any data are collected, ownership issues and the responsibilities that come with them need to be carefully worked out. Before undertaking any work, make sure you can answer the following questions:

✓ Who owns the data I am collecting?

✓ What rights do I have to publish the data?

✓ Does collecting these data impose any obligations on me?

 If you do not have firm answers for each of these questions, preferably in writing when financial interests are involved, you are not ready to begin your research.

It is also important to note that in most cases ownership provisions must be approved by the institution that receives and is responsible for the administration of research funds. Researchers therefore should not enter into agreements that affect the control and use of data without getting institutional approval. The results could be disastrous and expensive if ownership is disputed later.

6b. Data collection

There is no one best way to collect data. Different types of research call for different collection techniques. There are, however, four important considerations that apply to all data collection and that will help ensure the overall integrity of both the process and the information collected.

Appropriate methods. Reliable data are vitally dependent on reliable methods. If you use a test that can detect an effect in one of every 100 samples to find an effect that may not occur more frequently than 1 in every 1,000 cases, your results will not be reliable. Failure to find the effect could be due to either your experimental design or the lack of an effect, but you will not know which is true. The common saying, "garbage in, garbage out," applies to research methods.

Although the need for appropriate methods might seem obvious, studies have suggested that researchers sometimes use inappropriate statistical tests to evaluate their results (see articles by DeMets and Gardner, Additional Reading). Methods can also be compromised by bias—choosing one method or set of experimental conditions so that a particular conclusion can be drawn—or sloppy technique. Whatever the origin, the use of inappropriate methods in research compromises the integrity of research data and should be avoided. Responsible research is research conducted using appropriate, reliable methods.

Attention to detail. Quality research requires attention to detail. Experiments must be set up properly and the results accurately recorded, interpreted, and published. A failure to pay attention to detail can result in mistakes that will later have to be corrected and reported. Correcting the record takes time and resources that are better spent on the research itself.

Obviously, it is not possible to avoid all mistakes in research. However, take a look at the errata section of any scientific journal and ask yourself how the mistakes reported could have been avoided. Did the authors check to make sure that each figure was correctly labeled? Were the calculations double checked? Did someone check to make sure the authors were properly listed? Since others rely on their work, researchers have a responsibility to make sure their work is carefully undertaken and reported. Sloppy research wastes funds and should be avoided.

Authorized. Many types of data collection need to be authorized before they can proceed. Typically permission is needed to use:

✓ human and animal subjects in research;

✓ hazardous materials and biological agents;

✓ information contained in some libraries, databases, and archives;

✓ information posted on some Web sites;

✓ published photographs and other published information; and

✓ other copyrighted or patented processes or materials.

Researchers have a responsibility to know when permission is needed to collect or use specific data in their research. If you are not sure whether permission is needed, check before proceeding with data collection.

Recording. The final step in data collection is the physical process of recording the data in some type of notebook (hard copy), computer file (electronic copy), or other permanent "record" of the work done. The physical formats for recording data vary considerably, from measurements or observations to photographs or interview tapes. However data are recorded, it is important to keep in mind that the purpose of any record is to document what was actually done and the results that were achieved.

In recording data, keep two simple rules in mind to avoid problems later, should someone ask about or question your work:

✓ Hard-copy evidence should be entered into a numbered, bound notebook so that there is no question later about the date the experiment was run, the order in which the data were collected, or the results achieved. Do not use loose-leaf notebooks or simply collect pages of evidence in a file. Do not change records in a bound notebook without noting the date and reasons for the change.

✓ Electronic evidence should be validated in some way to assure that it was actually recorded on a particular date and not changed at some later date. It is easy to change dates on computers and thereby alter the date a particular file seems to have been created. If you collect your data electronically, you must be able to demonstrate that they are valid and have not been changed.

As you record your data, it may be helpful to think about them as the legal tender of research—the currency researchers cash in when they apply for grants, publish, are considered for promotion, and enter into business ventures. To have and hold their value, research data must be properly recorded.

6c. Data protection

Once collected, data must be properly protected. They may be needed later:

✓ to confirm research findings,

✓ to establish priority, or

✓ to be reanalyzed by other researchers.

Over time, data, as the currency of research, become an investment in research. If the data are not properly protected, the investment, whether public or private, could become worthless.

Data storage. The responsible handling of data begins with proper storage and protection from accidental damage, loss, or theft:

✓ Lab notebooks should be stored in a safe place.

✓ Computer files should be backed up and the backup data saved in a secure place that is physically removed from the original data.

✓ Samples should be appropriately saved so that they will not degrade over time.

✓ Care should be taken to reduce the risk of fire, flood, and other catastrophic events.

Properly store and protect your data. They are valuable.

Confidentiality. Some data are collected with the understanding that only authorized individuals will use them for specific purposes. In such cases, care needs to be taken to assure that privacy agreements are honored. This is particularly true of data that contain personal information that can be linked to specific individuals. It is also true of confidential information about protected processes and materials. If a company shares confidential data about a process with a researcher prior to seeking a patent on that process, the researcher must take care to make sure the data are kept confidential.

Data that are subject to privacy restrictions must be stored in a safe place that is accessible only to authorized personnel. Using random codes to identify individual subjects, rather than names or social security numbers, can also further protect private information. Access to these codes can then be restricted to provide a double layer of protection. Whatever the method used to protect private or confidential information, the researcher who collects or uses the information has the primary responsibility for its protection.

Period of retention. Data should be retained for a reasonable period of time to allow other researchers to check results or to use the data for other purposes. There is, however, no common definition of a *reasonable period of time.* NIH generally requires that data be retained for 3 years following the submission of the final financial report. Some government programs require retention for up to 7 years. A few universities have adopted data-retention policies that set specific time periods in the same range, that is, between 3 and 7 years. Aside from these specific guidelines, however, there is no comprehensive rule for data retention or, when called for, data destruction.

It is difficult to predict when data collected sometime in the past could be useful. When a new disease emerges, such as AIDS, researchers use stored samples/data to pinpoint first occurrences and the likely course of development of the disease. Although the original data were not stored for this purpose, they nonetheless can be useful for tracking diseases years later. Stored data are also useful for understanding social questions. The Department of Energy committee that made recommendations on appropriate compensation for improper human radiation experiments conducted during the Cold War pulled together data collected as far back as the 1950's. Researchers also cannot predict when someone will challenge their work and ask to see the original data.

Given the different reasons data could be useful over long periods of time, researchers should give some thought to retaining data longer than some minimum period required by specific regulations. How long is reasonable will vary from field to field and institution to institution. Nevertheless, it is important to have a clear retention policy that balances the best interests of society with those of the research institution and the individual researcher. Before throwing out notebooks, cleaning out files, or erasing your computer memory, give careful consideration to who might benefit from or ask to see your data in the future.

6d. Data sharing

It is widely agreed that research data should be shared, but deciding when and with whom raises questions that are sometimes difficult to answer.

Researchers are not expected to and in most instances should not release preliminary data, that is, data that have not been carefully checked and validated. The one exception to this rule would be preliminary data that could potentially benefit the public. A researcher who has strong preliminary indications of a major threat to public health, such as unexpected side effects from a drug or an unrecognized environmental health problem, may have good reason to

NIH Data Sharing Policy and Implementation Guidance
(Updated: March 5, 2003)

Goals of Sharing Data

Data sharing promotes many goals of the NIH research endeavor. It is particularly important for unique data that cannot be readily replicated. Data sharing allows scientists to expedite the translation of research results into knowledge, products, and procedures to improve human health.

There are many reasons to share data from NIH-supported studies. Sharing data reinforces open scientific inquiry, encourages diversity of analysis and opinion, promotes new research, makes possible the testing of new or alternative hypotheses and methods of analysis, supports studies on data collection methods and measurement, facilitates the education of new researchers, enables the exploration of topics not envisioned by the initial investigators, and permits the creation of new datasets when data from multiple sources are combined.

In NIH's view, all data should be considered for data sharing. **Data should be made as widely and freely available as possible while safeguarding the privacy of participants, and protecting confidential and proprietary data.** To facilitate data sharing, investigators submitting a research application requesting $500,000 or more of direct costs in any single year to NIH on or after October 1, 2003, are expected to include a plan for sharing final research data for research purposes, or state why data sharing is not possible.

http://grants1.nih.gov/grants/policy/data_sharing/data_sharing_guidance.htm

share this information with the public and other researchers before it is fully validated. Data that have no immediate public benefit, such as the discovery of a basic scientific process that could eventually lead to public benefits, in most instances is best held until the researcher is confident that the results will stand.

Researchers can withhold confirmed or validated data until they have had time to establish their priority for their work through publication or, in rare cases, a public announcement. They do not have to release data on a day-to-day or experiment-to-experiment basis for other researchers to use, even though this might speed the advance of knowledge. Provided no agreements have been made to the contrary, keeping data confidential prior to publication is a commonly accepted practice that most researchers and funding agencies accept.

Once a researcher has published the results of an experiment, it is generally expected that all the information about that experiment, including the final data, should be freely available for other researchers to check and use. Some journals formally require that the data published in articles be available to other researchers upon request or stored in public databases. In the specific case of federally funded research that is used in setting policies that have the effect of law, research data must be made available in response to Freedom of Information Act (FOIA) requests (OMB, Circular A-110). There is, in other words, considerable support for sharing data with other researchers and the public unless there are compelling reasons for confidentiality.

6e. Future considerations

The continued evolution of data policies will likely be driven by a number of different issues, including the growing complexity of data and debates about proper control.

Complexity. Our capacity to generate data sometimes outstrips our capacity to store and share it. Data storage and sharing were major problems during the early years of the Human Genome project. They continue to pose problems for any research area that is able to generate massive amounts of information efficiently and inexpensively. DNA microarray chips can generate 10,000 bits of information with a single, easily conducted test. The logistics of storing and sharing this information presents a monumental challenge for everyone engaged in research. Even when researchers want to, it is not always clear how they should go about collecting, storing, and sharing data responsibly.

Control. In large projects, questions frequently arise about the control of data, particularly when financial interests are at stake. Should researchers participating in large,

Research Committee, Society for Academic Emergency Medicine
Guidelines for Clinical Investigator Involvement in
Industry-sponsored Clinical Trials

IV. Trial Data Management

1. The industry sponsor and the investigators should have a firm commitment to thorough monitoring of the trial at every step.

2. All data collected in the trial should be open to scrutiny by both the investigators and the industry sponsor.

3. Clinical investigators should have substantial input into the initial analytic plan and also any subsequent amendments that occur during the trial period.

4. When possible, statistical analysis of the data should be conducted by an entity independent of the researchers and the sponsor. For trials using interim analysis, use of an independent entity is particularly important. Decisions to prematurely stop a trial should be based upon predetermined criteria.

5. Consideration should be given to the use of an unbiased, blinded "clinical evaluation committee" for trials that involve assessment of potentially subjective endpoints.

6. The industry sponsors must share the results of all data analyses with the principal investigators. Selective withholding or incomplete reporting of data analyses to the principal investigators is unacceptable.

7. Trial results and data analysis should be shared with the principal investigators as soon as they become available. Delays by the industry sponsors for marketing or related purposes are unacceptable.

http://www.saem.org/download/edward.pdf

multi-site clinical trials have the right to publish their own findings, that is, retain some control over their own data, or should the collection, storage, and interpretation be centralized? This issue is currently unresolved and the subject of intense public debate.

National security. Recent events have heightened concerns about the possible use of data from publicly supported research by terrorists and nations that could pose a threat to national security. Efforts are underway to address these concerns through voluntary policies and new

Federal regulations (e.g., USA Patriot Act of 2001) that will assure reasonable control without unduly restricting the ability of researchers to share their work and ideas freely with one another (see the recent report, *Biological Threats and Terrorism,* Additional Reading). Researchers whose work could be affected by these concerns should keep abreast of ongoing policy development and regulation.

However these issues are resolved, researchers have been the most important component of responsible data management practices in the past and will likely remain so as long as the public feels the majority of researchers can be trusted. With this in mind, ask yourself how someone funding your research would feel if he or she had a chance to take a close look at your data management practices.

Questions for discussion

1 Should research data belong to researchers rather than to research institutions?

2 Should data recording practices be standardized to facilitate sharing and monitoring? What recording practices could be standardized?

3 What interpretation practices could be standardized? How does your laboratory verify the accuracy and validity of data before its disclosure or use in grant proposals and publications?

4 Who should pay the cost of sharing data? Who should have access to the data?

5 How long should researchers be able to withhold data to allow time to protect ownership claims? How long should research data be stored?

Resources

Policies, Reports, and Policy Statements

American Statistical Association. *Ethical Guidelines for Statistical Practice*, Alexandria, VA: American Statistical Association, 1999. (available at: http://www.amstat.org/profession/index.cfm?fuseacti on=ethicalstatistics/)

Council on Government Relations. *Policy Considerations: Access to and Retention of Research Data*, Washington, D.C.: 1995. (available at: http://206.151.87.67/docs/ DataRetentionIntroduction.htm)

Food and Drug Administration. *Good Laboratory Practices for Designing Toxicology Studies for Petition Submissions and Notifications*, 21 CFR Part 58 (2002). (available at: http://www. cfsan.fda.gov/~dms/opa-pt58.html)

Harvard University, Office of Technology Licensing. *Record-Keeping Procedures*, 2000. (available at: http://www.otd. harvard.edu/inventions/ip/patents/recordkeeping/)

National Institutes of Health. *NIH Data Sharing Policy and Implementation Guidance*, 2003. (available at: http://grants1.nih. gov/grants/policy/data_sharing/data_sharing_guidance.htm)

Society for Clinical Data Management. *Good Clinical Data Management Practices*, Version 2, Hillsborough, NJ: Society for Clinical Data Management, 2002. (available at: https://www.scdm. org/GCDMP/Default.asp)

United States. Congress. *USA Patriot Act of 2001*, PL 107-56, 2001. (available at: http://frwebgate.access.gpo.gov/cgi-bin/getdoc. cgi?dbname=107_cong_public_laws&docid=f:publ056.107.pdf)

University of Pittsburgh. *Guidelines on Data Retention and Access*, Pittsburgh, PA: University of Pittsburgh, 1997. (available at: http://www.pitt.edu/~provost/retention.html)

General Information Web Sites

National Institutes of Health. Office of Extramural Research. *NIH Data Sharing Policy*, Washington, DC: National Institutes of Health. http://grants.nih.gov/grants/policy/data_sharing/

Society for Clinical Data Management. *Home Page*. http://www.scdm. org/

Additional Reading

Campbell, EG, Clarridge, BR, Gokhale, M, Birenbaum, L, Hilgartner, S, Holtzman, NA, Blumenthal, D. "Data Withholding in Academic Genetics: Evidence from a National Survey," *Journal of the American Medical Association* 287, 4 (2002): 473-480.

Council on Government Relations. *Materials Transfer in Academia*, Washington, DC: Council on Government Relations, 1997. DeMets, DL. "Statistics and Ethics in Medical Research," *Science and Engineering Ethics* 5, 1 (1999): 97-111.

Gardner, MJ. "An Exploratory Study of Statistical Assessment of Papers Published in the British Medical Journal," *Journal of the American Medical Association* 263, March 10 (1990): 1355-1357.

Kanare, HM. *Writing the Laboratory Notebook*, Washington, DC: American Chemical Society, 1985.

Knobler, SL, Mahmoud, AAF, Pray, LA, eds. *Biological Threats and Terrorism: Assessing the Science and Response Capabilities: Workshop Summary*. Washington, DC: National Academy Press, 2002.

Stevens, AR. *Ownership and Retention of Data*, Washington, DC: National Association of College and University Attorneys, 1997.

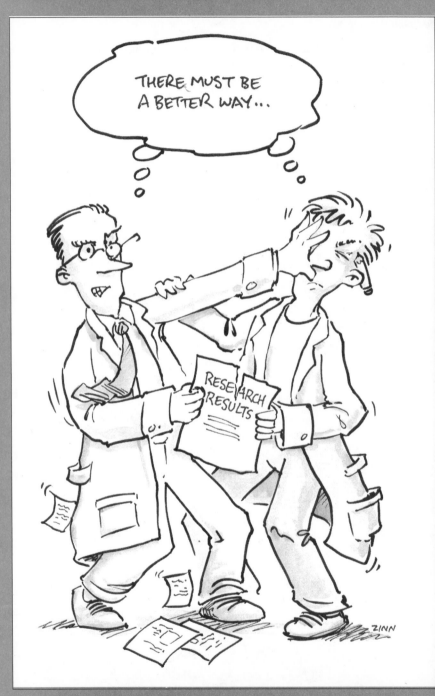

Mentor-trainee working relationships?

7. Mentor and Trainee Responsibilities

While conducting investigations, researchers often assume the added role of mentors to trainees.* The mentor-trainee relationship is complex and brings into play potential conflicts. How much time—training time for the mentor, research time for the trainee—should each devote to the other? Who gets credit for ideas that take shape during the course of a shared experiment? Who *owns* the results? When does a trainee become an *independent researcher?*

The essential elements of a productive mentor-trainee relationship are difficult to codify into rules or guidelines,

Case Study

At a recent meeting, several faculty in a large, research-oriented science department raised concerns about their mentoring program. While mindful of the many demands they all faced, they wondered whether changes were needed in the way the department assigned, trained, and oversaw mentors. The ensuing discussion raised some potentially good suggestions, which most agreed were best referred to a special committee for further discussion and recommendations. With a little arm twisting, Susan D., an advanced graduate student; Dr. Linda L., a postdoc; and Dr. Bill K., an established researcher, were recruited to serve.

At their first meeting, the three colleagues quickly agreed to tackle first the question of goals. If they knew what mentoring was expected to achieve, they could then assess the strengths and weaknesses of their current program and make suggestions for change. With this settled, they decided to spend some time talking with their peers and then get back together to compare notes. When they met the next time:

What goals would you expect each member of the committee to recommend?

Why might different members of the committee recommend different goals?

Assuming they came to the conclusion that some improvements were needed, what avenues are open to change the way mentors and trainees interact?

---

* The term "trainee" is used in this chapter to refer to anyone learning to be a researcher under an established researcher's supervision. This includes principally graduate students and postdoctoral fellows (postdocs), but may also include undergraduate and high school students working on research projects or junior research faculty, research scientists, and research staff.

leaving most of the decisions about responsible mentoring to the individuals involved. Common sense suggests that good mentoring should begin with:

✓ a clear understanding of mutual responsibilities,

✓ a commitment to maintain a productive and supportive research environment,

✓ proper supervision and review, and

✓ an understanding that the main purpose of the relationship is to prepare trainees to become successful researchers.

Understandings and agreements, however, will count for little if they are not backed up by firm commitments to make a relationship work.

Knowing the importance of personal commitments, researchers should carefully consider what responsibilities they have to trainees before they take on the essential task of training new researchers. Trainees, in turn, should be we aware of their responsibilities to mentors before accepting a position in a laboratory or program.

7a. Basic responsibilities

Mentor-trainee relationships begin when an experienced and an inexperienced researcher agree to work together. Each brings something to the table under such an arrangement. The experienced researcher has knowledge and skills that the inexperienced researcher needs to learn. She or he may also provide support for the trainee's research and education. Inexperienced researchers, whether graduate student, postdoctoral student (postdoc), research staff, or junior researcher, provide labor and fresh ideas. Under a productive relationship, the two work together to advance knowledge and put ideas to work. When the relationship breaks down, it is often because one of the parties is not getting from the relationship what she or he expected.

National Academy of Sciences
On Being a Mentor to Students in Science and Engineering

What is a Mentor?

In the broad sense intended here, a mentor is someone who takes a special interest in helping another person develop into a successful professional. Some students, particularly those working in large laboratories and institutions, find it difficult to develop a close relationship with their faculty adviser or laboratory director. They might have to find their mentor elsewhere—perhaps a fellow student, another faculty member, a wise friend, or another person with experience who offers continuing guidance and support.

In the realm of science and engineering, we might say that a good mentor seeks to help a student optimize an educational experience, to assist the student's socialization into a disciplinary culture, and to help the student find suitable employment. These obligations can extend well beyond formal schooling and continue into or through the student's career.

http://www.nap.edu/readingroom/books/mentor/

One way to avoid problems is to establish basic under-standings about important issues early in the relationship. Trainees need to know:

✓ how much time they will be expected to spend on their mentor's research;

✓ the criteria that will be used for judging performance and form the basis of letters of recommendation;

✓ how responsibilities are shared or divided in the research setting;

✓ standard operating procedures, such as the way data are recorded and interpreted; and, most importantly,

✓ how credit is assigned, that is, how authorship and ownership are established.

Clarifying these issues early in a mentor-trainee relationship can prevent problems from arising later.

The need for early understanding is not one sided. Mentors need to know that a trainee will:

✓ do assigned work in a conscientious way,

✓ respect the authority of others working in the research setting,

✓ follow research regulations and research protocols, and

✓ live by agreements established for authorship and ownership.

Mentors invest time and resources in trainees. Trainees should respect this time and use resources responsibly, keeping their mentors informed about changing research interests or other circumstances that could affect their work.

A Guide to Training and Mentoring in the Intramural Research Program at NIH

A mentor is a person who has achieved career success and counsels and guides another for the purpose of helping him or her achieve like success. Research supervisors should always be mentors; they have the responsibility to discuss with and advise a trainee on aspects of his or her work and professional development. The trainee may find additional mentors informally—or the training institution may designate them. They are very important in the overall experience of the trainee and may contribute to research productivity as well....

Training in the skills of mentorship itself is important, especially for those who plan careers in research or teaching. Postdoctoral trainees should learn to train and guide others, for example, by working with more junior individuals, supervising technical staff, or training students. The characteristics considered important by a fellow in selecting a supervisor and other mentors—interest in contributing to the career development of another scientist, research accomplishments, professional networking, accessibility, and past success cultivating the professional development of fellows—are characteristics that trainees may eventually strive to emulate in their own careers.

Although this Section has emphasized the responsibilities of supervisors and others in research institutions to provide mentoring to trainees to facilitate their professional development, trainees also have responsibilities. Collaborative research frequently requires productive interactions among fellows themselves as well as recognition of their roles as part of a team effort. In addition, fellows must have a commitment to the work of the laboratory and Institute and to the achievement of their goals. They cannot be passive participants in their training; they should appropriately make known their satisfactions, dissatisfactions, and needs clearly and often.

http://www1.od.nih.gov/oir/sourcebook/ethic-conduct/mentor-guide.htm

Arriving at basic understandings early in a mentor-trainee relationship is not easy, given the unequal power relationship between them. Mentors are in a position to lay out expectations, but it can be difficult for a trainee to raise questions early in a relationship about credit and authorship practices. To avoid putting trainees in the awkward position of having to raise these issues, mentors should be prepared to take the lead in raising issues that are of concern to the trainee as well as those that are of interest to the mentor. Developing written guidance on a laboratory's authorship and publication practices should also be considered.

7b. Research environment

Different mentors establish different research environments. Some laboratories are highly competitive; others emphasize cooperation. Some mentors are intimately involved in all aspects of the projects they supervise; others delegate authority. Similarly, different researchers like to work in different environments. Some enjoy independence; others like to have close working relationships with colleagues. Some thrive in competitive environments; others prefer cooperative working relationships. Although there is no single formula for a "good" research environment, there are some fundamentals that mentors and trainees should keep in mind.

Equal treatment. Research ability is not tied to race, gender, ethnicity, or sexual orientation. These factors have no bearing on one's success as a researcher. Therefore, research environments should not put someone at a disadvantage based on who they are. If competition is encouraged in a way that puts any distinguishable group at a significant disadvantage, it is not acceptable. All students should be subject to the same level of supervision and scrutiny. Aside from legal obligations to avoid discrimination in the workplace, researchers have a

University of Michigan
Mentoring within a Diverse Community

Need for Role Models

Students from historically underrepresented or marginalized groups have a harder time finding faculty role models who might have had experiences similar to their own. As some students say, they want to find "someone who looks like me;" "someone who immediately understands my experiences and perspectives;" "someone whose very presence lets me know I, too, can make it in the academy."

Feelings of Isolation

Students from historically underrepresented groups can feel particularly isolated or alienated from other students in their departments, especially if the composition of a program is highly homogenous.

Burden of Being a Spokesperson

Students from underrepresented groups often expend a lot of time and energy speaking up when issues such as race, class, gender, or sexual orientation arise or are being ignored. These students point out how most of their peers have an advantage in not carrying such a burden.

Seeking Balance

Students observe that professors need to devote large parts of their lives to their work in order to be successful in the academy. Students from all disciplines tell us that they feel faculty expect them to spend every waking minute on their work. This perception of faculty expectations, accurate or not, is of grave concern to students who have children or wish to, as well as for those who want to balance their lives with their other interests.

http://www.rackham.umich.edu/StudentInfo/Publications/FacultyMentoring/contents.html

professional obligation to work to assure equal access to their profession, particularly if their work is publicly supported.

Professional practice. Researchers should maintain research environments that respect accepted practices for the responsible conduct of research. Trainees learn by example as well as formal training. They assume, not unreasonably, that the practices they observe are *appropriate* practices. Mentors therefore have an obligation to maintain research environments that set appropriate examples. They should not themselves make unreasonable authorship demands, fail to honor agreements made with trainees, inappropriately cut corners in research, or engage in other practices that run counter to accepted practices for the responsible conduct of research.

Training in the responsible conduct of research. Beginning in 1989 and in line with recommendations made by the Institute of Medicine (IOM, 1989), the National Institutes of Health (NIH) required recipients of National Research Service Institutional Training Program awards (training grants) to offer instruction in the responsible conduct of research (RCR). The National Science Foundation (NSF) has a similar requirement for recipients of its Integrative Graduate Education and Research Traineeship (IGERT) Program awards. Later reports, notably by the 1995 Commission on Research Integrity, called for broadening this requirement to all PHS-funded research, but such a requirement has not been implemented. Nonetheless, there is widespread agreement that RCR training should be integral to the research environment, with heavy emphasis given to the role the mentor plays in providing this training.

7c. Supervision and review

When mentors accept trainees, they assume responsibility for assuring that the persons under their supervision are appropriately and properly trained. This responsibility is particularly important in research since for the most part there are no other checks on the qualifications of new researchers. Researchers do not take licensing exams. They are judged primarily by the quality of their research, which should be best known to the person directly supervising their work, that is, to their mentor.

Proper supervision of a trainee takes time. In one way or another a mentor needs to:

✓ assure proper instruction in research methods,

✓ foster the intellectual development of the trainee,

✓ impart an understanding of responsible research practices, and

✓ routinely check to make sure the trainee develops into a responsible researcher.

Mentors do not need to check all aspects of a trainee's work directly. In large laboratories, postdocs often supervise graduate students and laboratory technicians might teach specific laboratory skills. Training in the responsible use of animals is often done through an animal care program. However, the ultimate responsibility for training rests with the mentor.

Proper supervision and review play an important role in quality control. Trainees can make mistakes. Some have deliberately falsified or fabricated data. Mentors should review work done under their supervision carefully enough to assure that it is well done and accurate. This can be accomplished by:

Emory University School of Medicine
Policy for Postdoctoral Fellows

Mentor Obligations

Postdoctoral research opportunities at Emory University School of Medicine are intended to foster the training of basic and clinical research scientists. Included within this goal is the concept that postdoctoral fellows, with the guidance of their mentors, will develop a scientific project that utilizes the creativity and independence of the fellow. In this spirit, the mentor will provide adequate facilities, funds, and the appropriate guidance to achieve the agreed-upon goals of the project. In addition, mentors should provide guidance in critical review of scientific information, grant writing, manuscript writing and preparation, presentation of scientific information, and in the art of performing research. Mentors should also advise and as possible, aid fellows in decisions regarding future employment potential and career paths. Mentor review of fellow performance and career development should be conducted at least once per year. A member(s) of the departmental senior faculty should be designated to serve as liaison with departmental post-doctoral fellows, faculty, and the Office of Postdoctoral Education and its advisory committees.

http://www.med.emory.edu/POSTDOC/Web%20Forms/Adobe%20Forms/Policy%20for%20Post doctoral%20Fellows%207.1.05-1.pdf

✓ reviewing laboratory notebooks and other compilations of data;

✓ reading manuscripts prepared by trainees carefully to assure that they are accurate, well-reasoned, and give proper credit to others;

✓ meeting with trainees on a regular basis to keep in touch with the work they are doing; and

✓ encouraging trainees to present and discuss data at laboratory meetings.

Some of this responsibility can be delegated to others, but as with all other matters regarding training, the mentor should assume ultimate responsibility.

7d. Transition to independent researcher

The ultimate goal of research training is to produce independent researchers who can establish their own research programs, take on trainees, and help research-dependent disciplines grow. This means that the mentor's final responsibility to trainees is to help them get established as independent researchers.

History has repeatedly shown that experienced researchers often do not give over control to the next generation easily. They have a difficult time seeing ideas they planted grow in another person or having someone they trained head out in new directions. And yet in many fields, it is well documented that researchers are most productive early in their careers, when they are first making their way as independent researchers.

The problem of trainee versus independent researcher is most apparent in postdoctoral training. Postdocs, as they are commonly known, are usually well prepared to undertake independent work, and yet they are still working under someone else's supervision. The fact that they are neither official students nor official faculty gives them few rights and protections. The fact that they are usually supported by someone else's funding leaves them open to exploitation. To protect against such exploitation, a new organization, the National Postdoctoral Association, has recently been established "to address national issues relevant to postdocs and focus public debate on how to improve the lives of postdocs at all levels."

Researchers who supervise postdocs should carefully work out their relationship with this unique and important group of researchers in training. Some supervision is still necessary, but not as much as for graduate students. Postdocs may have their own funding and assume all the duties of a principal investigator, even if for administrative purposes their funding comes through their mentor. They may deserve first authorship on all of their papers, even though the mentor was involved in the research. Most importantly, they should be encouraged to develop the independence and record needed to get a regular research appointment, thereby paying back society's investment in years of research training and the student's investment in her or his own career.

Questions for discussion

1.   Can elements of the mentor-trainee relationship be reduced to a written agreement that both parties would sign at the beginning of the relationship?

2.   What are the qualities of a good mentor? A good trainee?

3.   What are the qualities of a good research environment and how can they be fostered?

4.   What is the purpose of postdoctoral training and how long should it last?

5.   Can good mentoring be taught, monitored, and evaluated?

Resources

Policies, Reports, and Policy Statements

Commission on Research Integrity. *Integrity and Misconduct in Research: Report of the Commission on Research Integrity,* Washington, DC: Health and Human Services, 1995. (available at: http://ori.hhs.gov/documents/report_commission.pdf)

Gottesman, MM. *A Guide to Training and Mentoring in the Intramural Research Program at NIH,* Bethesda, MD: National Institutes of Health, 1999. (available at: http://www1.od.nih.gov/oir/sourcebook/ethic-conduct/mentor-guide.htm)

Institute of Medicine. *The Responsible Conduct of Research in the Health Sciences,* Washington, DC: National Academies of Science, 1989. (available at: http://search.nap.edu/books/0309062373/html/)

National Institutes of Health. Alcohol, Drug, and Mental Health Administration. "Requirement for Programs on the Responsible Conduct of Research in National Research Service Award Institutional Training Programs," *NIH Guide for Grants and Contracts* 18 (1989): 1. (available at: http://grants.nih.gov/grants/guide/historical/1989_12_22_Vol_18_No_45.pdf)

National Science Foundation. *Integrative Graduate Education and Research Traineeship (IGERT) Program,* Washington, DC: NSF, 2002. (available at: http://www.nsf.gov/pubs/2002/nsf02145/nsf02145.pdf)

General Information Web Sites

Association for Women in Science. *Home Page.* http://www.awis.org/

MentorNet. *The E-Mentoring Network for Women in Engineering and Science.* http://www.mentornet.net/

National Postdoctoral Association. Home Page. (available at: http://www.nationalpostdoc.org/site/c.eoJMIWOBIrH/b.1388059/k.DBBE/NPA_Home.htm)

Additional Reading

Association for Women in Science. *Mentoring Means Future Scientists*, Washington, DC: Association for Women in Science, 1993.

Gadlin, H, Jessar, K. "Preempting Discord: Prenuptial Agreements for Scientists," *The NIH Catalyst*, May-June (2002). (available at: http://ori.hhs.gov/education/preempting_discord.shtml)

National Academy of Sciences, National Academy of Engineering, Institute of Medicine. *Adviser, Teacher, Role Model, Friend: On Being a Mentor to Students in Science and Engineering*, Washington, DC: National Academy Press, 1997. (available at: http://www.nap.edu/readingroom/books/mentor/)

University of Michigan. Horace H. Rackham School of Graduate Studies. *How to Mentor Graduate Students: A Guide for Faculty in a Diverse University*, Ann Arbor, MI: University of Michigan, 2002. (available at: http://www.rackham.umich.edu/StudentInfo/Publications/FacultyMentoring/contents.html)

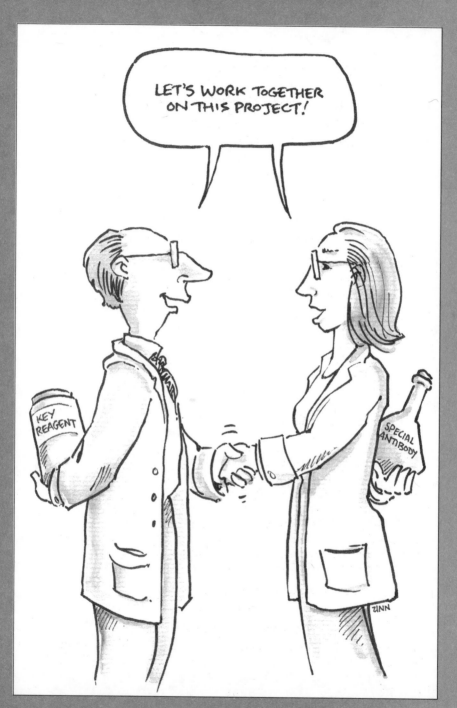

Collaboration or competition?

8. Collaborative Research

Researchers increasingly collaborate with colleagues who have the expertise and/or resources needed to carry out a particular project. Collaborations can be as simple as one researcher sharing reagents or techniques with another researcher. They can be as complex as multi-centered clinical trials that involve academic research centers, private hospitals, and for-profit companies studying thousands of patients in different states or even countries.

Any project that has more than one person working on it requires some collaboration, i.e., working together. In most projects, however, one person, commonly called the "principal investigator" or PI, is in charge. Others work under the PI's direction. In this chapter, the focus will be on groups of researchers who are all more or less equal partners working on a common, "collaborative" project.

In collaborative projects, researchers continue to have the responsibilities discussed in other chapters in the *ORI*

Case Study

Sharon, Ben, and Terra met during a late-night discussion at a professional meeting. They share a common interest in learning disorders but come from different scientific backgrounds. Sharon works at the cutting edge of brain imaging technology. Ben is an educational psychologist interested in pre-school children in inner cities. Terra has been putting her knowledge as a physiologist to work exploring the effects of alternative medicines.

As late night turns to early morning, the newly met trio begins to see benefits from working together and starts sketching out a grant proposal. The scientific ideas quickly fall into place, but some of the logistics raise questions that need answers.

Who should submit the proposal, through which university?

Do all three need to get IRB approval to work on the project?

What will happen if their work has practical applications?

How should they go about answering these questions? Are there other important questions that should be asked as well?

Introduction to RCR, but they assume some additional responsibilities stemming from collaborative relationships. These additional responsibilities arise from the added burdens of:

✓ the increasingly complex roles and relationships;

✓ common, but not necessarily identical, interests;

✓ management requirements; and

✓ cultural differences

inherent in any large project but especially in collaborative projects. Special attention to these added burdens can help keep collaborative projects running smoothly.

8a. Roles and relationships

Effective collaboration begins with a clear understanding of roles and relationships, which should begin the day the collaboration is established by discussing and reaching agreement on the details of the collaborative relations. Before any work is undertaken, there should be some common understanding of:

✓ the goals of the project and anticipated outcomes;

✓ the role each partner in the collaboration will play;

✓ how data will be collected, stored, and shared;

✓ how changes in the research design will be made;

✓ who will be responsible for drafting publications;

✓ the criteria that will be used to identify and rank contributing authors;

✓ who will be responsible for submitting reports and meeting other requirements;

✓ who will be responsible for or have the authority to speak publicly for the collaboration;

✓ how intellectual property rights and ownership issues will be resolved; and

✓ how the collaboration can be changed and when it will come to an end.

Clear understandings in advance are the best way to avoid complications and disagreements later in a collaboration.

Obviously, situations can arise during a collaboration that could not have been anticipated in advance. For this reason, it is important for effective communication to continue throughout any collaborative project. Collaborators should:

✓ share findings with colleagues in the collaboration and pay attention to what others are doing;

✓ report and discuss problems as well as findings;

✓ make other collaborators aware of any important changes, such as changes in key personnel; and

✓ share related news and developments so that everyone in the collaboration is equally knowledgeable about important information.

All of these points may seem obvious, but they can easily get lost in the day-to-day details of doing research. However, if you are working with collaborators, keep in touch. Without effective communication, collaborations can easily run into problems and dissolve.

8b. Management

In addition to effective communication, collaborative projects should have effective management plans that cover:

✓ financial issues,

✓ training and supervision,

✓ formal agreements, and

✓ compliance.

When a PI is in charge of all of the work done on a project, the lines of responsibility are clear. The PI is ultimately responsible for all aspects of the project, from financial expenditures to staff training, data collection, reporting, and wrapping up the project. In collaborative research, the partners in the collaboration share responsibilities. Under these circumstances, an effective management plan is essential.

Financial management. The expenditure of Federal research funds is subject to financial management rules issued by the Office of Management and Budget in Circulars A-21 and A-110 (see boxes, below and next page). A-21 covers all aspects of financial management, from accounting procedures to reporting requirements. For example, one section carefully describes, in fairly technical terms, allowable and unallowable expenses. Some travel costs are allowed; others are not. A-110 sets out rules for issuing government grants and contracts. It explains how equipment should be purchased and used, even after the project has come to an end.

Office of Management and Budget Circular A-21

48. Travel costs.

a. **General.** Travel costs are the expenses for transportation, lodging, subsistence, and related items incurred by employees who are in travel status on official business of the institution. Such costs may be charged on an actual basis, on a per diem or mileage basis in lieu of actual costs incurred, or on a combination of the two, provided the method used is applied to an entire trip and not to selected days of the trip, results in reasonable charges, and is in accordance with the institution's travel policy and practices consistently applied to all institutional travel activities.

b. **Lodging and subsistence.** Costs incurred by employees and officers for travel, including costs of lodging, other subsistence, and incidental expenses, shall be considered reasonable and allowable only to the extent such costs do not exceed charges normally allowed by the institution in its regular operations as a result of an institutional policy and the amounts claimed under sponsored agreements represent reasonable and allocable costs.

c. **Commercial air travel.** Airfare costs in excess of the lowest available commercial discount airfare....

http://www.whitehouse.gov/omb/circulars/a021/a021.html

Office of Management and Budget
Circular A-110

34. Equipment.

(c) The recipient shall use the equipment in the project or program for which it was acquired as long as needed, whether or not the project or program continues to be supported by Federal funds and shall not encumber the property without approval of the Federal awarding agency. When no longer needed for the original project or program, the recipient shall use the equipment in connection with its other federally-sponsored activities, in the following order of priority: (i) Activities sponsored by the Federal awarding agency which funded the original project, then (ii) activities sponsored by other Federal awarding agencies.

http://www.whitehouse.gov/omb/circulars/a110/a110.html

Every federally funded research project must adhere to the rules set out in A-21 and A-110. Therefore, collaborative projects must be managed in ways that assure that all expenditures are in compliance, from those incurred by the primary investigators working at major research institutions to survey workers or clinicians working in the field.

Training and supervision. Wherever they work, research staff should be properly trained and supervised. In some instances the training is mandatory. Anyone who works with research animals or human subjects must have formal training. The same is true of staff who work with hazardous substances or biohazards. These requirements extend to everyone working on a collaborative project, whether they are at a different institution, in another state, or even another country. Management plans for collaborative projects therefore should include the training and supervision of all researchers and staff working on the project.

Formal agreements. Some aspects of collaborative projects must be worked out in advance in formal agreements. For example, when research is carried out in more than one place, it is sometimes necessary to transfer materials from one institution to another. Since many materials are carefully controlled, to protect either safety or ownership, the terms of transfer should be carefully spelled out, including (see NIH-recommended provisions below):

✓ who owns the materials,

✓ the use to which they can be put, and

✓ proper acknowledgment of the source.

These agreements help protect the interests of the collaborators by assuring that ownership will be respected and that the materials will be properly used.

Compliance. Increasingly, research institutions must in one way or another certify that they are in compliance with specific research regulations. When research institutions are involved in collaborative projects, an institution's responsibility for compliance can extend to other institutions. If the other institution is a U.S. university with a large

National Institutes of Health
Recommended Provisions for a Materials Transfer Letter

1. The [supplied] MATERIAL is the property of the PROVIDER and is made available as a service to the research community.

2. THIS MATERIAL IS NOT FOR USE IN HUMAN SUBJECTS.

3. The MATERIAL will be used for teaching or not-for-profit research purposes only.

4. The MATERIAL will not be further distributed to others without the PROVIDER's written consent....

6. Any MATERIAL delivered pursuant to this Agreement is understood to be experimental in nature and may have hazardous properties....

7. The RECIPIENT agrees to use the MATERIAL in compliance with all applicable statutes and regulations.

8. The MATERIAL is provided at no cost, or with an optional transmittal fee solely to reimburse the PROVIDER for its preparation and distribution costs. If a fee is requested, the amount will be indicated here: [insert fee]

http://www.ott.nih.gov/pdfs/MTA.pdf

research portfolio, that institution most likely already has a compliance plan in place. However, if the other institution does not do a great deal of research or is located in another country, it may not have thought about its compliance responsibilities. Management plans for collaborative projects must take into account the need for meeting compliance responsibilities throughout the project sites and not just at one institution.

8c. Different research settings

Most researchers devote their careers to one field of research and spend their time talking with colleagues with similar interests. However, science is increasingly best served when researchers work with colleagues in other fields. Physicians and engineers have teamed together to develop miniature wireless devices that can gather information while passing normally through the body. Computer scientists are working with organic chemists and biologists to develop faster computers and more flexible display devices. Collaborative projects encourage researchers to pursue interdisciplinary research.

For the most part, interdisciplinary research follows the same rules and practices as disciplinary research. There are times, however, when researchers in different fields bring different practices or expectations to a project. When this happens, researchers might think of adopting two common-sense rules:

✓ do not ignore any responsibilities, and

✓ when there are choices about appropriate action, select the most demanding option.

When in doubt, it makes sense to seek the highest rather than the lowest denominator.

Different expectations can enter a project in a number of ways, especially when judgments about responsible practice are involved. The government and some research institutions allow researchers to earn up to $10,000 through consulting or other outside employment before they have to declare a potential conflict of interest (discussed in Chapter 5). Others institutions use lower thresholds, in some cases requiring researchers to report conflicts of interest if they have any outside financial interests. Different institutions also manage conflicts of interest in different ways, from supervision or reporting to outright prohibition. When there are differences in reporting policy, the prudent course of action is to go with the lowest financial threshold and accept the most stringent management plan, even though some researchers working on the collaborative project may not be required to do so.

Ownership issues also raise questions about which rules to follow. One party to a collaboration may have no interest in reporting a promising idea for development; another may feel under an obligation to do so, following either a university's or Federal policy. There may also be different understandings among the different institutions that are part of a collaboration about what constitutes disclosable information and who owns the information once it is disclosed. Given the consequences of disputes that can erupt in these situations, it is essential that every collaborative project settle disclosure and ownership issues early in the project before disputes arise. Waiting longer opens the door for misunderstandings and disputed claims when one of the parties in the collaboration makes a valuable discovery.

Finally, there are significant differences in the way researchers in different fields and even different laboratories carry out the routine business of collecting data and publishing results. Some still collect data in bound laboratory notebooks; others use computers. In some fields, it is common practice to circulate early results in newsletters and/or abstracts; in other fields, journal publications are the preferred mode of communication. Different fields have different ways and standards for listing authors. These and other differences should be addressed openly and early in any collaboration to assure that misunderstandings do not arise later over data collection and publication.

Questions for discussion

1. Why should collaborative research be encouraged?

2. When should research collaborations be formalized?

3. Are there any drawbacks to collaborative research? What problems can they raise?

4. Which country's rules should be used in collaborative projects that are carried out in different countries?

5. What steps should be taken when a collaborative project comes to an end or a collaboration is dissolved?

Resources

Policies, Reports, and Policy Statements

National Institutes of Health. "Principles And Guidelines for Recipients of NIH Research Grants and Contracts on Obtaining and Disseminating Biomedical Research Resources: Final Notice," *64 FR 72090* (1999). (available at: http://www.ott.nih.gov/pdfs/64FR72090.pdf)

Office of Management and Budget. *OMB Circular A-110, Uniform Administrative Requirements for Grants and Other Agreements with Institutions of Higher Education, Hospitals and Other Non-Profit Organizations*, Washington, DC: OMB, 1999. (available at: http://www.whitehouse.gov/omb/circulars/a110/a110.html)

————. *Circular A-21: Cost Principles for Educational Institutions*, Washington, DC: OMB, 2000. (available at http://www.whitehouse.gov/omb/circulars/a021/a021.html)

Additional Reading

Davis, TP, ed. *Management of Biomedical Research Laboratories: Proceedings of a National Conference*, Tucson, AZ: University of Arizona, 1998. (available at: http://ori.hhs.gov/conferences/past_conf.shtml)

Gadlin, H, Jessar, K. "Preempting Discord: Prenuptial Agreements for Scientists," *The NIH Catalyst*, May-June (2002). (available at: http://ori.hhs.gov/education/preempt_discord.shtml)

Gottesman, MM. *Funding of Intramural Research Program/ Extramural Research Program Collaborations*, 1999. (available at: http://www1.od.nih.gov/oir/sourcebook/ethic-conduct/fund-irp-erp-3-00.htm)

Government-University-Industry Research Roundtable, NetLibrary Inc. *Overcoming Barriers to Collaborative Research: Report of a Workshop*, Washington, DC: National Academy Press, 1999.

Macrina, FL. *Dynamic Issues in Scientific Integrity: Collaborative Research*, Washington, DC: American Society for Microbiology, 1995. (available at: http://www.asm.org/ASM/files/ CCLIBRARYFILES/FILENAME/0000000841/research.pdf)

Schwartz, J. *Silence is not Golden: Making Collaborations Work*, Bethesda, MD: National Institutes of Health, nd. (available at: http://ori.hhs.gov/education/science_not_golden.shtml)

Vonortas, NS, Hamdi, M. *United Nations Conference on Trade and Development. Partnerships and Networking in Science and Technology for Development*, New York: United Nations, 2002.

Wagner, CS, United States. Office of Science and Technology Policy, Science and Technology Policy Institute (Rand Corporation). *Linking Effectively: Learning Lessons from Successful Collaboration in Science and Technology*, Santa Monica, CA: Rand, 2002.

Part IV.

Reporting and
Reviewing
Research

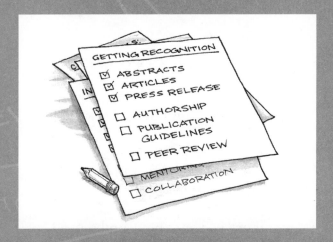

Part IV: Reporting and Reviewing Research

RESEARCH HAS NO VALUE IF IT IS NOT MADE

public. Results are shared with colleagues

so they can be tested, used to advance

knowledge, and put to work. They

are shared with the public and poli-

cymakers so that they can be used to

make decisions about funding and practical

application.

While researchers might engage in research simply for their own satisfaction, if their work receives public support, they have a responsibility to share that work with others.

Chapter 9, Authorship and Publication, covers the responsibilities researchers have when they share results with others through informal communications, oral presentations, scholarly publications, and public statements. Whatever mechanism is used, research results should be shared honestly, efficiently, and without bias. Dishonesty and bias undermine the usefulness of research publications; inefficiency (publishing the same research several times) wastes public funds and the valuable time of reviewers and journal editors.

Chapter 10, Peer Review, describes the responsibilities researchers have when they review the work of other researchers. Non-peers—individuals who do not have equal training and knowledge—cannot evaluate the quality and importance of research. Peers can and therefore play a crucial role in many important decisions about the funding, publication, and use of research.

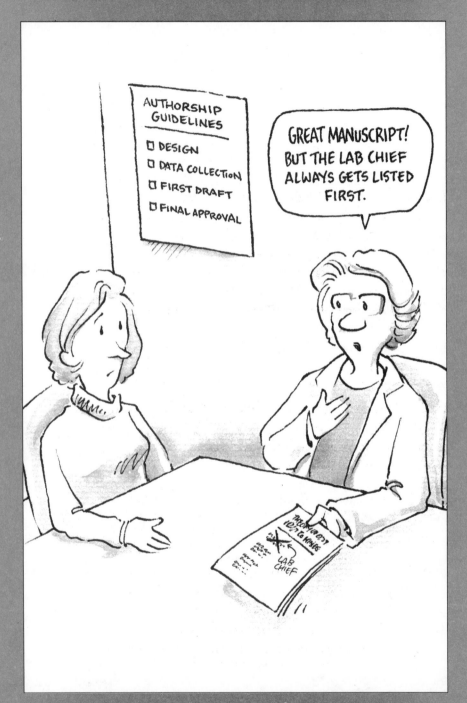

Responsible authorship?

9. Authorship and Publication

Researchers share the results of their works with colleagues and the public in a variety of ways. Early results are usually shared during laboratory meetings, in seminars, and at professional meetings. Final results are usually communicated to others through scholarly articles and books. Public communication takes place through press releases, public announcements, newspaper articles, and public testimony. Some of these ways of communicating research results (i.e., of publication) are well structured and controlled; others are informal and have few controls.

Whether structured or informal, controlled or free ranging, responsible publication in research should ideally meet some minimum standards. All forms of publication should present:

Case Study

As his first major grant is coming to an end, several important elements of Dr. Sanjay K.'s research suddenly fall into place. The last series of experiments his graduate student ran clearly link the gene they are studying to a particular type of cancer. His postdoc's work on the proteins associated with this gene could pave the way for possible cures. With these results in hand, he is finally ready to make a strong case for continued support and, happily, his pending promotion. All he has to do now is publish the results.

A week later, Sanjay's optimism starts to fade. As might have been expected, his department chair was delighted with his progress, but then suggested that the first paper announcing the results come out under her name to give it broader circulation. Meanwhile, his postdoc and graduate student have gotten into a heated debate about the order their names should appear on the paper; the university's public affairs office has asked for a summary of the results for a press release; and the technology transfer office has called telling him to hold all publications until they can evaluate the commercial potential of his work.

What should Sanjay do?

Which of these problems should Sanjay tackle first?

Is there anything he could have done to assure that things went more smoothly when he was ready to publish his results?

✓ a full and fair description of the work undertaken,

✓ an accurate report of the results, and

✓ an honest and open assessment of the findings.

In assessing the completeness of any publications, researchers should ask whether they have described:

✓ what they did (methods),

✓ what they discovered (results), and

✓ what they make of their discovery (discussion).

It is, however, not as easy as one might anticipate to meet these expectations.

9a. Authorship

The names that appear at the beginning of a paper serve one important purpose. They let others know who conducted the research and should get credit for it. It is important to know who conducted the research in case there are questions about methods, data, and the interpretation of results. Likewise, the credit derived from publications is used to determine a researcher's worth. Researchers are valued and promoted in accordance with the quality and quantity of their research publications. Consequently, the authors listed on papers should fairly and accurately represent the person or persons responsible for the work in question.

Contribution. Authorship is generally limited to individuals who make significant contributions to the work that is reported. This includes anyone who:

✓ was intimately involved in the conception and design of the research,

✓ assumed responsibility for data collection and interpretation,

✓ participated in drafting the publication, and

✓ approved the final version of the publication.

There is disagreement, however, over whether authorship should be limited to individuals who contribute to all phases

ICJME Statement on Authorship

An "author" is generally considered to be someone who has made substantive intellectual contributions to a published study... .

Authorship credit should be based on 1) substantial contributions to conception and design, or acquisition of data, or analysis and interpretation of data; 2) drafting the article or revising it critically for important intellectual content; and 3) final approval of the version to be published. Authors should meet conditions 1, 2, and 3.

All persons designated as authors should qualify for authorship, and all those who qualify should be listed.

Each author should have participated sufficiently in the work to take public responsibility for appropriate portions of the content.

http://www.icmje.org/

of a publication or whether individuals who made more limited contributions deserve authorship credit.

The widely accepted *Uniform Requirements for Manuscripts Submitted to Biomedical Journals*, authored by the International Committee of Medical Journal Editors (ICMJE), sets a high standard for authorship. It recommends limiting authorship to persons who contribute to the conception and design of the work or to data collection and interpretation and, in addition, play an important role in drafting and approving the final publication. Anyone who plays a lesser role can be listed under *acknowledgments* but not at the beginning of the paper as an *author*.

As influential as they are, the ICMJE recommendations on authorship are not uniformly followed, even in journals that subscribe to the ICMJE *Requirements*. Practices for determining authors vary considerably by discipline and even from laboratory to laboratory. This places most of the responsibility for decisions about authorship on the researchers who participated in the work reported in each publication. These decisions are best made early in any project, to avoid misunderstandings and later disputes about authorship.

Importance. Authors are usually listed in their order of importance, with the designation *first* or *last author* carrying special weight, although practices again vary by discipline. Academic institutions usually will not promote researchers to the rank of tenured faculty until they have been listed as first or last author on one or more papers.

As with the principle of contribution, however, there are no clear rules for determining who should be listed as first author or the order in which other authors should be listed. The ICMJE *Requirements* simply note that:

> The order of authorship on the byline should be a joint decision of the coauthors. Authors should be prepared to explain the order in which authors are listed.

Some journals have specific rules for listing authors; others do not, again placing most of the responsibility for this decision on the authors themselves.

Corresponding or primary author. Many journals now require one author, called the *corresponding* or *primary* author, to assume responsibility for all aspects of a publication, including:

✓ the accuracy of the data,

✓ the names listed as authors (all deserve authorship and no one has been neglected),

✓ approval of the final draft by all authors, and

✓ handling all correspondence and responding to inquiries.

In accepting this responsibility, *corresponding authors* should take special note of the fact that they are acting on behalf of their colleagues. Any mistakes they make or fail to catch will affect their colleagues' as well as their own careers.

9b. Elements of a responsible publication

Each element of a publication serves an important purpose and must be carefully prepared to make sure it serves that purpose.

Abstracts. Abstracts summarize the content of publications in sufficient detail to allow other researchers to assess relevance to their own work. Abstracts, therefore, should neither understate nor overstate the importance of findings. Negative results that might be important to other researchers or the public should be mentioned. The data presented in the abstract should be the same as the data presented in the body of the publication—an obvious requirement, but one that studies of publication practices show some authors do not follow (see Pitkin, Additional Reading).

Standards for Reporting Research Results
The CONSORT Statement

Abstract

To comprehend the results of a randomized controlled trial (RCT), readers must understand its design, conduct, analysis, and interpretation. That goal can be achieved only through complete transparency from authors. Despite several decades of educational efforts, the reporting of RCTs needs improvement. Investigators and editors developed the original CONSORT (Consolidated Standards of Reporting Trials) statement to help authors improve reporting by using a checklist and flow diagram. The revised CONSORT statement presented here incorporates new evidence and addresses some criticisms of the original statement.

The checklist items pertain to the content of the Title, Abstract, Introduction, Methods, Results, and Discussion. The revised checklist includes 22 items selected because empirical evidence indicates that not reporting the information is associated with biased estimates of treatment effect, or because the information is essential to judge the reliability or relevance of the findings. We intended the flow diagram to depict the passage of participants through an RCT. The revised flow diagram depicts information from four stages of a trial (enrollment, intervention allocation, follow-up, and analysis). The diagram explicitly shows the number of participants, for each intervention group, included in the primary data analysis. Inclusion of these numbers allows the reader to judge whether the authors have done an intention-to-treat analysis.

http://www.consort-statement.org/Statement/revisedstatement.htm

To ensure completeness and accuracy, many journals now use *structured* abstracts. This assures that all of the key elements of the publication are mentioned and easily identified. With scientific publications now running in the millions per year in well over 100,000 journals, researchers cannot read all seemingly relevant publications in detail. They must rely on abstracts to point them to important developments and findings.

Methods. Researchers cannot check and build on the work of others without knowing how it was conducted. Methods therefore should be described in sufficient detail to allow other researchers to replicate them. When researchers use well-established methods, this section of a publication can be shortened, provided appropriate references are given to a full description of the methods along with any changes that have been made. New or unique methods should be described in more detail to allow other researchers to replicate the work.

Results. Research results should be reported in sufficient detail to allow other researchers to draw their own conclusions about the work. This does not mean that every piece of recorded data should be reported. Researchers can and must process their raw data before publication (to keep publications to a reasonable size if for no other reason). However, results should not be left out just because they do not agree with the conclusions the authors would like to reach. The results section should represent a complete summary of what was discovered, leaving interpretations for the closing discussion.

Discussion. Researchers can and should evaluate the significance of their findings under *discussion*—also called *conclusion* or *summary*. This portion of a publication helps those who are less familiar with the field understand the importance of the findings. It also provides a venue for identifying unresolved problems and future research needs.

Since the *discussion* is read by individuals who may not be able to evaluate its validity, it is particularly important that authors avoid bias and one-sided reporting in this section. Cautions and other interpretations should be mentioned along with the limitations of the study to provide a balanced view of the reported results. Review articles (articles that survey research findings in particular areas) should make an honest effort to cover all relevant work. It is not always easy to recognize one's own biases, which is a good reason to ask colleagues to read and comment on manuscripts before they are submitted for publication.

Notes, bibliography, and acknowledgments. Notes, bibliography, and acknowledgments should be used to place publications in context and to give credit to others for their ideas, support, and work. They serve to:

✓ provide support for important statements of fact or assumptions,

✓ document the work of others used in the publication,

✓ point to additional reading and resources, and

✓ recognize the support of funding agencies or colleagues and staff who do not qualify as authors.

Since others rely on and trust this information, it, along with every other element of a responsible publication, should be fair and accurate.

9c. Practices that should be avoided

Competition in research for funding and recognition places considerable pressure on researchers to publish. Ideally, quality should matter more than quantity, but in reality quantity—the number of articles published—is often used as a measure of productivity and ability. However, no matter how important it may be to publish, some publication practices should be avoided.

The Council of Science Editors
A New Standard for Authorship (1998 proposal)
Paul J. Friedman, MD

Publication has become the essential achievement for academic advancement for both clinical and basic scientists, although the type and number of publications demanded may vary widely. Despite a recent increased emphasis on teaching as a meritorious activity, faculty and trainees realistically feel intense pressure to publish. One unfortunate result has been a proliferation of papers and journals and a variety of abuses of trainees, junior colleagues, and patients, and of integrity.

To help restore a sense of proportion and confidence in the validity of biomedical publication, this conference proposes a new step in the evolution of the concept of authorship. We propose to publish the contributions of the individuals associated with a manuscript. The information will be solicited on a modified copyright form, which will be filled out and signed by all the authors. We propose a check-off list, such as the following:

☐ Concept	☐ Data collection and/or processing
☐ Design	☐ Analysis and/or interpretation
☐ Supervision	☐ Literature search
☐ Writing	☐ Critical review
☐ Resources	☐ Material

http://www.councilscienceeditors.org/services/friedman_article.cfm

Honorary authorship. The practice of listing undeserving authors on publications, called "honorary" authorship, is widely condemned and in the extreme considered by some to constitute a form of research misconduct. However, common agreement notwithstanding, honorary authorship is a significant problem in research publication today (see articles by Drenth and Flanagin, Additional Reading). Researchers are listed on publications because they:

✓ are the chair of the department or program in which the research was conducted,

✓ provided funding for the research,

✓ are the leading researcher in the area,

✓ provided reagents, or

✓ served as a mentor to the primary author.

Persons in these positions can make significant contributions (see left) to a publication and may deserve recognition. However, they should not be listed if these are the only contributions they made.

Salami publication. *Salami publication* (sometimes called bologna or trivial publication) is the practice of dividing one significant piece of research into a number of small experiments (least publishable units or LPUs), simply to increase the number of publications. This practice may distort the value of the work by increasing the number of studies that appear to support it. It also wastes valuable time and resources. Before an article is published it is reviewed, edited, and in one form or another prepared for publication. After publication it is entered into indexes and databases, such as the National Library of Medicine's *PubMed®*. Libraries and individuals purchase the journal in which it is published. If the same information could be summarized in one article as opposed to two, three, or more, everyone involved, from the publishers to libraries and the researchers who have to keep up to date on current information, benefits. Researchers therefore should avoid trivial or salami publication.

Duplicate publication. Duplicate publication is the practice of publishing the same information a second time without acknowledging the first publication. This practice not only wastes time and resources but can also distort the research record and endanger public health.

Researchers rely on meta-analyses (analyses of a group of similar experiments or *studies of studies*) to improve their understanding of difficult problems. One clinical trial or epidemiological study may not produce clear evidence, but the pooled results of many related studies can. However, if some of the studies in the pooled study (meta-analysis) have been published two or more times without proper notice, the results of the meta-analysis will be unfairly weighted in the direction of the duplicate publication. Therefore, duplicate publication is not only deceptive but poses real dangers to public health and safety (see articles by Jefferson and Tramer, Additional Reading).

Premature public statements. Academic or scholarly publication practices are designed to assure that the information conveyed to broader audiences through these practices is accurate and fairly presented. While the system is not foolproof and erroneous or biased information is from time to time published, standard publication practices do serve an important quality control role in research. Accordingly, researchers should follow standard publication practices when making research results public and not issue premature public statements about their work before it has been reviewed. From time to time there may be overriding circumstances, such as early indications of a significant threat to public health or safety, but for the most part research results should be made public only after they have been carefully reviewed and properly prepared for publication.

Questions for discussion

1 What are the accepted criteria for authorship in your field of research? If there are none, what should they be?

2 Should researchers be allowed to omit some details from the methods section of their publications until they have had time to patent their methods?

3 What should a researcher do if the journal that has accepted a publication will not let the researcher publish the method or results in as much detail as the researcher feels is necessary?

4 What should a researcher do if an undeserving author in a position of some authority demands authorship status on a paper?

5 What factors should be considered when making a decision to publish the results of a study in one article versus several articles?

Resources

Policies, Reports, and Policy Statements

Council of Biology Editors. *Scientific Style and Format*, CBE, 2006. (available at: http://www.councilscienceeditors.org/publications/style.cfm)

International Committee of Medical Journal Editors. *Uniform Requirements for Manuscripts Submitted to Biomedical Journals*, 2001. (available at: http://www.icmje.org/)

Michigan State University. *Michigan State University Guidelines on Authorship*, East Lansing, MI: MSU, 1998. (available at: http://www.msu.edu/unit/vprgs/authorshipguidelines.htm)

Society for Neuroscience. *Responsible Conduct Regarding Scientific Communication*, SN, 1996. (available at: http://www.sfn.org/index.cfm?pagename=responsibleConduct&section=publications)

Additional Reading

Begg, C, Cho, MK, Eastwood, S, Horton, R, Moher, D, Oking, I, Pitkin, RM, Rennie, D, Schulz, KF, Simel, D, Stroup, D. "Improving the Quality of Reporting of Randomized Controlled Trials: The CONSORT Statement," *Journal of the American Medical Association* 276 (1996): 637-639.

Bloemenkamp, DGM, Walvoort, HC, Hart, W, Overbeke, AJPM. "[Duplicate publication of articles in the Dutch Journal of Medicine in 1996]," *Nederlands Tijdschrift voor Geneeskunde* 143, 43 (1999): 2150-2153.

Budd, JM, Sievert, M, Schultz, TR. "Phenomena of Retraction: Reasons for Retraction and Citations to the Publications," *Journal of the American Medical Association* 280, 3 (1998): 296-297.

Budd, JM, Sievert, M, Schultz, TR, Scoville, C. "Effects of Article Retraction on Citation and Practice in Medicine," *Bulletin of the Medical Libraries Association* 87, 4 (1999): 437-443.

Drenth, JP. "Multiple Authorship: The Contribution of Senior Authors," *Journal of the American Medical Association* 280, 3 (1998): 219-221.

Flanagin, A, Carey, LA, Fontanarosa, PB, Phillips, SG, Pace, BP, Lundberg, GD, Rennie, D. "Prevalence of Articles with Honorary Authors and Ghost Authors in Peer-reviewed Medical Journals," *Journal of the American Medical Association* 280, 3 (1998): 222-224.

Hoen, WP, Walvoort, HC, Overbeke, AJ. "What are the Factors Determining Authorship and the Order of the Authors' Names? A Study Among Authors of the Nederlands Tijdschrift voor Geneeskunde (Dutch Journal of Medicine)," *Journal of the American Medical Association* 280, 3 (1998): 217-218.

Jadad, AR, Cook, DJ, Jones, A, Klassen, TP, Tugwell, P, Moher, M, Moher, D. "Methodology and Reports of Systematic Reviews and Meta-analyses: A Comparison of Cochrane Reviews with Articles Published in Paper-based Journals," *Journal of the American Medical Association* 280, 3 (1998): 278-280.

Jefferson, T. "Redundant Publication in Biomedical Sciences: Scientific Misconduct or Necessity?" *Science and Engineering Ethics* 4, 2 (1998): 135-140.

Jones, AH, McLellan, F. *Ethical Issues in Biomedical Publication*, Baltimore: Johns Hopkins University Press, 2000.

Pitkin, RM, Branagan, MA. "Can the Accuracy of Abstracts be Improved by Providing Specific Instructions? A Randomized Controlled Trial," *Journal of the American Medical Association* 280, 3 (1998): 267-269.

Pitkin, RM, Branagan, MA, Burmeister, LF. "Accuracy of Data in Abstracts of Published Research Articles," *Journal of the American Medical Association* 281, 12 (1999): 1129-1130.

Scherer, RW, Crawley, B. "Reporting of Randomized Clinical Trial Descriptors and Use of Structured Abstracts," *Journal of the American Medical Association* 280, 3 (1998): 269-272.

Speck, BW. *Publication Peer Review: An Annotated Bibliography, Bibliographies and Indexes in Mass Media and Communications, no. 7*, Westport, CT: Greenwood Press, 1993.

Tarnow, E. "The Authorship List in Science: Junior Physicists' Perceptions of Who Appears and Why," *Science and Engineering Ethics* 5, 1 (1999): 73-88.

Tramer, MR, Reynolds, DJ, Moore, RA, McQuay, HJ. "Impact of Covert Duplicate Publication on Meta-analysis: A Case Study," *British Medical Journal* 315, 7109 (1997): 635-640.

Wilcox, LJ. "Authorship: The Coin of the Realm, The Source of Complaints," *Journal of the American Medical Association* 280, 3 (1998): 216-217.

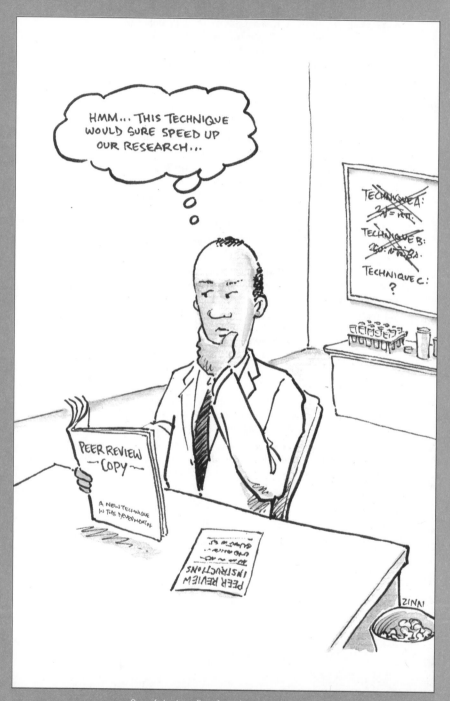

One of the benefits of serving as a peer reviewer?

10. Peer Review

Peer review—evaluation by colleagues with similar knowledge and experience—is an essential component of research and the self-regulation of professions. The average person does not have the knowledge and experience needed to assess the quality and importance of research. Peers do. Therefore many important decisions about research depend on advice from peers, including:

✓ which projects to fund (grant reviews),

✓ which research findings to publish (manuscript reviews),

✓ which scholars to hire and promote (personnel reviews), and

✓ which research is reliable (literature reviews and expert testimony).

The quality of the decisions made in each case depends heavily on the quality of peer review.

Case Study

Dr. Sung L. is struggling with the decision whether to agree to review the work of an advanced graduate student at another university for publication in the major journal in his field. He is familiar with the student's work and attended a session several months ago at which she presented a brief report on her work. It clearly overlaps with his research in a number of ways, which is one reason he has been asked to serve as a reviewer.

Dr. L. knows he is qualified to do the review and is confident he can provide an objective, constructive judgment of the students's work. However, since his students are working on similar problems, he is concerned about the appearance of a conflict of interest. In addition, he is not sure he wants to learn more about the work in question until he publishes his own work, to avoid later charges that he unfairly used some of the student's ideas. Finally, there is the matter of yet another lost weekend doing the review, when his department chair has already told him to cut down on unpaid professional service.

Should Dr. L. agree to do the review?

If he is uncertain about his responsibilities, where can he get advice?

Would the situation be different if he had been asked to review the student's work for an appointment or promotion decision?

Peer review can make or break professional careers and directly influence public policy. The fate of entire research programs, health initiatives, or environmental and safety regulations can rest on peer assessment of proposed or completed research projects. For peer review to work, it must be:

✓ timely,

✓ thorough,

✓ constructive,

✓ free from personal bias, and

✓ respectful of the need for confidentiality.

Researchers who serve as peer reviewers should be mindful of the public as well as the professional consequences of their evaluations and exercise special care when making these evaluations.

10a. Meeting deadlines

The effort researchers put into peer review is for the most part not compensated. Researchers may receive reimbursement for travel and per diem when they attend special grant-review sessions and occasionally are paid a basic daily stipend, but this seldom covers the true cost of reviewing a manuscript or a stack of grant applications. As uncompensated effort, the time researchers devote to peer review can easily take second place to other obligations. Running a crucial experiment or submitting a grant application on time understandably is more important than reviewing someone else's work.

However pressed you are for time, if you agree to do a review, you should find the time to meet your obligation in a timely manner. Research is competitive. Researchers are rewarded for discoveries. They should not lose their priority for a discovery due to the tardiness of a reviewer sending comments on a manuscript. Research is also useful. The

Editors of the Publications Division
American Chemical Society

Ethical Obligations of Reviewers of Manuscripts

1. ...every scientist has an obligation to do a fair share of reviewing.

2. A chosen reviewer who feels inadequately qualified to judge the research reported in a manuscript should return it promptly to the editor.

3. A reviewer (or referee) of a manuscript should judge objectively the quality of the manuscript, of its experimental and theoretical work, of its interpretations and its exposition, with due regard to the maintenance of high scientific and literary standards. A reviewer should respect the intellectual independence of the authors.

4. A reviewer should be sensitive to the appearance of a conflict of interest....

6. A reviewer should treat a manuscript sent for review as a confidential document....

7. Reviewers should explain and support their judgments adequately....

8. A reviewer should be alert to failure of authors to cite relevant work by other scientists,...

9. A reviewer should act promptly, submitting a report in a timely manner.

10. Reviewers should not use or disclose unpublished information, arguments, or interpretations contained in a manuscript under consideration, except with the consent of the author....

http://pubs.acs.org/ethics/eg_ethic2000.pdf

announcement of discoveries that can benefit the public should not be delayed because someone who agreed to review a manuscript does not have the time to do the review.

Editors, program managers, and others who rely on peer review to make decisions generally provide a deadline for getting the review done when they first contact reviewers. Anyone who agrees to take on a peer review assignment under these conditions should meet the proposed deadline. If the time frame is not reasonable, either decline to do the review or ask for more time in advance. Do not delay someone else's work just because you are short on time.

10b. Assessing quality

Journal editors, grant administrators, and others rely on peers to assess the quality of proposed and published research. Some parts of an application or manuscript can be checked fairly easily. Are the calculations correct? Is the method that has been used or proposed appropriate? Do the reported results support the conclusions? Other parts are more difficult to confirm. Have the data been accurately recorded and reported? Were the experiments run? Did the subjects give consent? Do the articles cited in the references and bibliography contain the information they are said to contain?

Peers who are asked to make judgments about the quality of a proposed or completed project must do their best to determine whether the work they have been asked to review is internally consistent and conforms to the practices of their field of research. This certainly includes:

✓ assessing whether the research methods are appropriate;

✓ checking calculations and/or confirming the logic of important arguments;

✓ making sure the conclusions are supported by the evidence presented; and

✓ confirming that the relevant literature has been consulted and cited.

At the very least, peer reviewers should be expected to assess whether the manuscript or proposal under review makes sense and conforms to accepted practices, based on the information presented.

Research that conforms to accepted practices can still have problems. Research quality can be compromised by:

✓ careless mistakes made in reporting data and/or listing citations;

✓ the deliberate fabrication and falsification of data;

✓ improper use of material by others (plagiarism);

✓ inaccurate reporting of conflicts of interest, contributors/
authors; and

✓ the failure to mention important prior work, either by others
or by the researcher submitting a paper for publication.

However, how much peer reviewers can or should do to
detect these and other deceptive or sloppy practices
remains subject to debate.

There are limits to the amount of checking that is both
reasonable and practical. Unless given permission to do so,
reviewers should not discuss the work they are reviewing
with the authors. In many cases, reviews are "blind" (no
author identification), so reviewers could not check with

Society for Neuroscience
Responsible Conduct Regarding Scientific Communication (1998)

2.   Reviewers of Manuscripts

2.1. Thorough scientific review is in the interest of the scientific community.

2.2. A thorough review must include consideration of the ethical dimensions of a
manuscript as well as its scientific merit.

2.3. All scientists are encouraged to participate if possible when asked to review a
manuscript.

2.4. Anonymity of reviewers should be preserved unless otherwise stated in the guidelines
for authors and for reviewers, or unless a reviewer requests disclosure.

2.5. Reviewers should be chosen for their high qualifications and objectivity regarding a
particular manuscript.

2.6. Reviews should not contain harsh language or personal attacks.

2.7. Reviews should be prompt as well as thorough.

2.8. Reviewers must not use non-public information contained in a manuscript to advance
their own research or financial interests.

2.9. Information contained in a manuscript under review is confidential and must not be
shared with others.

http://www.sfn.org/index.cfm?pagename = responsibleConduct_reviewersOfManuscripts/

authors even if they wanted to. In addition, it is not reasonable to expect reviewers to check every reference and detail. The fact remains, however, that peer reviewers frequently miss problems that might have been detected had the reviewer checked a little more carefully.

If you agree to serve as a peer reviewer, remember that you have essentially been asked to provide your stamp of approval for someone else's work. In such circumstances, it is wise to do your homework. Do not give your stamp of approval too easily.

10c. Judging importance

In addition to quality, peer reviewers are also asked to make judgments about the importance of proposed or published research. They are asked to answer questions such as:

✓ Assuming a researcher could carry out a proposed research project, is it important to do so?

✓ Are these research results important enough to publish?

✓ Has a researcher made important contributions to a field of study?

✓ Is this evidence important enough to be used in setting policy?

Along with quality, judgments about importance essentially determine which research is funded or published and which researchers are hired and relied upon for advice.

Peer reviewers do not always make judgments about importance with an open mind. Studies have shown that they can be swayed by:

✓ the stature of the researcher who conducted the research or the institution at which the research was conducted;

✓ country of origin;

✓ a preference for one research method over another, e.g., a clinical versus a laboratory approach; and

✓ the outcome of the studies under review.

For the most part, these factors should not have a bearing on judgments about importance and yet they do. Each has been shown to influence the judgments peer reviewers make about the publication of research results (see articles by Callaham, Cho, Dickersin, Godlee, Jadad, and Link, Additional Reading).

There is no simple solution to the problem of bias in peer review. Peers frequently are not of one mind about what is or is not important. One reviewer may feel that a field of research should move in one direction, a second in an entirely different direction. Often, it takes time and more research to find out whether a line of investigation or a particular set of findings is *important*. Nonetheless, researchers can take steps to lessen the impact of bias on their judgments and to help others judge for themselves whether a researcher has biases.

One way to lessen the impact of bias is to write *transparent* reviews. By "transparent" is meant laying out clearly for anyone reading the review how it was prepared, the literature that was used, and the reviewer's own possible biases. If reviewers fully and carefully explain how their judgments about importance were made, others can assess whether they want to accept those judgments.

A second way that has been proposed to lessen the impact of bias is to eliminate anonymous reviews. Some argue that this would lessen the candor and rigor of reviews; others that it would make reviewers more accountable. For the present, most reviews are anonymous, which places the burden for fairness on the reviewer. If you have strong feelings about a person or particular line of investigation, tell the person who asked you to do the review and consider whether you can, in fact, provide an impartial assessment.

10d. Preserving confidentiality

Some information that is shared during peer review is shared confidentially, that is, with the understanding that it will not be shared with anyone else without permission. Confidentiality is generally required during:

✓ grant reviews,

✓ manuscript reviews, and

✓ personnel reviews.

During grant and manuscript reviews, confidentiality helps protect ideas before they are funded or published. In personnel reviews, confidentiality is important to protect personal privacy.

Peer reviewers have an obligation to preserve confidentiality during the review process if they have been asked to do so. While this obligation might seem obvious, it can be compromised in some seemingly harmless and other more harmful ways. For example, although researchers sometimes do, it is *not acceptable* to do any of the following without getting permission:

✓ ask students or anyone else to conduct a review you were asked to do;

✓ use an idea or information contained in a grant proposal or unpublished manuscript before it becomes publicly available;

✓ discuss grant proposals or manuscripts you are reviewing with colleagues in your department or at a professional meeting;

✓ retain a copy of the reviewed material (generally manuscripts and grant proposals should be shredded or returned after the review is complete); and

✓ discuss personnel and hiring decisions with colleagues who are not part of the review process.

There may be times when some added advice during a review may be helpful, but reviewers should not seek this advice without getting permission. It may also be tempting to use information in a grant application or manuscript to speed up your own research, but until it has been made public, confidential information is not available for use, even to reviewers. If you are not comfortable protecting confidential information, then do not agree to be a peer reviewer.

Researchers who are in a position to pass judgment on the work of colleagues have significant power. They can hasten or slow that work; credit or discredit it. They have the power to shape entire fields of research and to influence public policy. If you have that power, make sure you use it responsibly and with some compassion, knowing that what you say and do directly affects the careers of other researchers.

Questions for discussion

1. What should researchers or students do if a colleague or mentor asks them to take a look at a manuscript they have not been authorized to review?

2. What information contained in a manuscript or proposal should reviewers be expected to check?

3. Should peer review be anonymous?

4. How can researchers who sit on committees that advise on research directions separate their own interests from the best interests of the field they are helping shape?

5. What would happen if the public lost confidence in peer review and looked for other mechanisms to judge the quality and importance of research?

Resources

Policies, Reports, and Policy Statements

International Committee of Medical Journal Editors. *Uniform Requirements for Manuscripts Submitted to Biomedical Journals*, 2006. (available at: http://www.icmje.org/)

National Institutes of Health. *NIH Guide – Objectivity in Research*, Bethesda, MD: NIH, 1995. (available at: http://grants2.nih.gov/grants/guide/notice-files/not95-179.html)

University of Michigan Medical School. *Guidelines for the Responsible Conduct of Research: Right and Responsibilities of Peer Review*, Ann Arbor, MI: UM, 1999. (available at: http://www.responsibility.research.umich.edu/UMMSpeer.html)

General Information Web Sites

International Congress on Peer Review and Biomedical Publication. *Home Page*, 2005. http://www.ama-assn.org/public/peer/peerhome.htm

Office of Extramural Research. National Institutes of Health. OER: *Peer Review Policy and Issues*, 2003. http://grants1.nih.gov/grants/peer/peer.htm

Additional Reading

Armstrong, JS. "Peer Review for Journals: Evidence on Quality Control, Fairness, and Innovation," *Science and Engineering Ethics* 3, 1 (1997): 63-84.

Black, N, van Rooyen, S, Godlee, F, Smith, R, Evans, S. "What Makes a Good Reviewer and a Good Review for a General Medical Journal?" *Journal of the American Medical Association* 280, 3 (1998): 231-233.

Callaham, ML, Baxt, WG, Waeckerle, JF, Wears, RL. "Reliability of Editors' Subjective Quality Ratings of Peer Reviews of Manuscripts," *Journal of the American Medical Association* 280, 3 (1998): 229-231.

Callaham, ML, Wears, RL, Weber, EJ, Barton, C, Young, G. "Positive-outcome Bias and Other Limitations in the Outcome of Research Abstracts Submitted to a Scientific Meeting," *Journal of the American Medical Association* 280, 3 (1998): 254-7.

Cho, MK, Justice, AC, Winker, MA, Berlin, JA, Waeckerle, JF, Callaham, ML, Rennie, D. "Masking Author Identity in Peer Review: What Factors Influence Masking Success?" *Journal of the American Medical Association* 280, 3 (1998): 243-245.

Dickersin, K. "How Important is Publication Bias? A Synthesis of Available Data," *AIDS Education and Prevention* 9, 1 Suppl (1997): 15-21.

Dickersin, K, Fredman, L, Flegal, KM, Scott, JD, Crawley, B. "Is There a Sex Bias in Choosing Editors? Epidemiology Journals as an Example," *Journal of the American Medical Association* 280, 3 (1998): 260-264.

Evans, A, McNutt, R, Fletcher, S, Fletcher, R. "The Characteristics of Peer Reviewers Who Produce Good-quality Reviews," *Journal of General Internal Medicine* 8, August 8 (1993): 422-428.

Fletcher, RH, Fletcher, SW. "Evidence for the Effectiveness of Peer Review," *Science and Engineering Ethics* 3, 1 (1997): 35-50.

Godlee, F, Gale, CR, Martyn, CN. "Effect on the Quality of Peer Review of Blinding Reviewers and Asking Them to Sign Their Reports: A Randomized Controlled Trial," *Journal of the American Medical Association* 280, 3 (1998): 237-240.

Jadad, AR, Cook, DJ, Jones, A, Klassen, TP, Tugwell, P, Moher, M, and Moher, D. "Methodology and Reports of Systematic Reviews and Meta-Analyses: A Comparison of Cochrane Reviews with Articles Published in Paper-Based Journals." *Journal of the American Medical Association* 280, 3 (1998): 278-280.

Jefferson, T. *Peer Review in the Health Sciences*, London: British Medical Journal Books, 1999.

Justice, AC, Cho, MK, Winker, MA, Berlin, JA, Rennie, D. "Does Masking Author Identity Improve Peer Review Quality? A Randomized Controlled Trial," *Journal of the American Medical Association* 280, 3 (1998): 240-242.

Link, AM. "US and Non-US Submissions: An Analysis of Reviewer Bias," *Journal of the American Medical Association* 280, 3 (1998): 246-247.

Pitkin, RM, Branagan, MA, Burmeister, LF. "Effectiveness of a Journal Intervention to Improve Abstract Quality," *Journal of the American Medical Association* 283, 4 (2000): 481.

van Rooyen, S, Godlee, F, Evans, S, Black, N, Smith, R. "Effect of Open Peer Review on Quality of Reviews and on Reviewers' Recommendations: A Randomised Trial," *British Medical Journal* 318, 7175 (1999): 23-27.

van Rooyen, S, Godlee, F, Evans, S, Smith, R, Black, N. "Effect of Blinding and Unmasking on the Quality of Peer Review: A Randomized Trial," *Journal of the American Medical Association* 280, 3 (1998): 234-237.

———. "Effect of Blinding and Unmasking on the Quality of Peer Review," *Journal of General Internal Medicine* 14, 10 (1999): 622-624.

Part V.

Safe Driving and Responsible Research

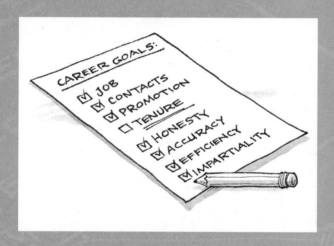

Part V: Safe Driving and Responsible Research

IT IS NOT EASY TO GO THROUGH LIFE DOING

everything we must or should do all of

the time. It should therefore come

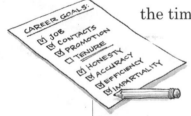

as no surprise that in many

small and some significant

ways, researchers do not always follow the

rules of the road for responsible conduct in

research. They roll through stop signs when

they clean up their data more than they

should, accept honorary authorship, purchase something with grant funds that is not strictly allowed, or give colleagues more favorable reviews than they deserve. From time to time, they drive faster than the posted speeds to arrive at their destination—a grant, a publication, new knowledge—a little more quickly.

We ignore *musts* and *shoulds* in life for different reasons. For one, society sends mixed messages about obeying rules. Should you turn in someone for cheating or "mind your own business"? Rules also can conflict with one another. Should you report misconduct if doing so puts your career at risk? And finally, we are amazingly adept at "bending" or "stretching" the rules by thinking up good reasons why a questionable course of action is acceptable under a particular set of circumstances, that is, at justifying our actions, whatever they are.

The ease with which rules can be bent or ignored is particularly evident early in the career track the majority of researchers traditionally follows. Studies consistently suggest that well over half and probably closer to three-quarters of college students cheat during their undergraduate years. In two separate studies, 1 in 10 research trainees reported a willingness to break the rules to get grants funded or papers published. Roughly the same number of students applying for research fellowships and residencies in medicine significantly misrepresents their research publications on résumés, as confirmed in studies conducted in six medical specialties. Presumably most individuals who cheat or inflate résumés know that it is wrong to do so, but they nonetheless find reason for engaging in these practices.

The same patterns of behavior can easily spill over into other aspects of research. The pressures that prompt students to bend or ignore the rules do not disappear after graduation. Getting into good schools is replaced by getting a good job and promotions. Competition for grades is replaced by competition to get funded and published. Too little time to study for tests is replaced by too little time to teach, mentor, provide service, and do research. The stakes may even increase later in careers, as family responsibilities are added into the mix and personal ambitions grow, making it even easier to put more pressure on the accelerator to get to your destination a little faster.

There are many quick-and-easy reasons that can be called up to justify bending or ignoring some of the rules of the road for responsible research:

✓ I already have enough information to know what the results will be, so there is no need to run the controls again, even though they did not give me the expected results the first time.

✓ No one funds truly exploratory research, so the only way to test new ideas is to use funds from an existing grant, even though these funds are for other work.

✓ If my bosses read my research papers rather than counting them, I wouldn't have to publish the same research twice or chop it up into small, insignificant pieces.

✓ Given the competition in this field, you cut your own throat if you share your methods and information with colleagues too freely.

✓ They will cut off my funds if I report these results, so for the good of my laboratory and staff I should sit on them for a while longer.

✓ I know my research is not going to harm anyone, so why waste my time and the time of the IRB getting permission.

Rules are not always reasonable or rationally applied. Life and colleagues are not always fair. Good guys do sometimes seem to come in last.

However, the problem with quick-and-easy justifications and catchy phrases is they fail to take into consideration the larger consequences of our actions. What would happen if everyone decided, for one "good" reason or another, to run stop signs, drive on the wrong side of the road, or ignore the speed limit? Obviously, chaos would quickly ensue and driving would no longer be safe (or become even more hazardous than it is already). The same would be true of research if researchers routinely ignored responsible research practices and did what they thought was necessary simply to achieve some end, whether the discovery of truth, the development of something useful, or personal success.

As stated at the beginning of the *ORI Introduction to RCR*, there is no one best way to undertake research, no universal method that applies to all scientific investigations. Accepted practices for the responsible conduct of research can and do vary from discipline to discipline and even laboratory to laboratory. There are, however, some important shared values for the responsible conduct of research that bind all researchers together, including honesty, accuracy, efficiency, and objectivity. There are no excuses for compromising these values. Their central role in research is the responsibility of each and every researcher. Drive safely and be a responsible researcher.

Resources

Additional Reading

Baker, DR, Jackson, VP. "Misrepresentation of Publications by Radiology Residency Applicants," *Academic Radiology* 7, 9 (2000): 727-729.

Bilge, A, Shugerman, RP, Robertson, WO. "Misrepresentation of Authorship by Applicants to Pediatrics Training Programs," *Academic Medicine* 73, 5 (1998): 532-533.

Brown, S, Kalichman, MW. "Effects of Training in the Responsible Conduct of Research: A Survey of Graduate Students in Experimental Sciences," *Science and Engineering Ethics* 4, 4 (1998): 487-498.

Dale, JA, Schmitt, CM, Crosby, LA. "Misrepresentation of Research Criteria by Orthopaedic Residency Applicants," *Journal of Bone and Joint Surgery* 81, 12 (1999): 1679-1681.

Eastwood, S, Derish, P, Leash, E, Ordway, S. "Ethical Issues in Biomedical Research: Perceptions and Practices of Postdoctoral Research Fellows Responding to a Survey," *Science and Engineering Ethics* 2, 1 (1996): 89-114.

Goe, LC, Herrera, AM, Mower, WR. "Misrepresentation of Research Citations among Medical School Faculty Applicants," *Academic Medicine* 73, 11 (1998): 1183-1186.

Grover, M, Dharamshi, F, Goveia, C. "Deception by Applicants to Family Practice Residencies," *Family Medicine* 33, 6 (2001): 441-446.

Gurudevan, SV, Mower, WR. "Misrepresentation of Research Publications among Emergency Medicine Residency Applicants," *Annals of Emergency Medicine* 27, 3 (1996): 327-330.

Kalichman, MW, Friedman, PJ. "A Pilot Study of Biomedical Trainees' Perceptions Concerning Research Ethics," *Academic Medicine* 67, 11 (1992): 769-775.

McAlister, WP, Velyvis, JH, Uhl, RL. "Misrepresentation of Research Criteria by Orthopaedic Residency Applicants," *Journal of Bone and Joint Surgery* 82-A, 10 (2000): 1512-1513.

Panicek, DM, Schwartz, LH, Dershaw, DD, Ercolani, MC, Castellino, RA. "Misrepresentation of Publications by Applicants for Radiology Fellowships: Is It a Problem?" *American Journal of Roentgenology* 170, 3 (1998): 577-581.

Patel, MV, Pradhan, BB, Meals, RA. "Misrepresentation of Research Publications among Orthopedic Surgery Fellowship Applicants: A Comparison with Documented Misrepresentations in Other Fields," *Spine* 28, 7 (2003): 632-636; discussion 31.

Sekas, G, Hutson, WR. "Misrepresentation of Academic Accomplishments by Applicants for Gastroenterology Fellowships," *Annals of Internal Medicine* 123, 1 (1995): 38-41.

Notes

Notes